C0-AYJ-245

Hepatitis C, The Silent Epidemic

The Authoritative Guide

Hepatitis C, The Silent Epidemic

The Authoritative Guide

FRED K. ASKARI, M.D., PH.D.

Illustrations by
DANIEL S. CUTLER, C.M.I.

KLUWER ACADEMIC / PLENUM PUBLISHERS
NEW YORK, BOSTON, DORDRECHT, LONDON, MOSCOW

3 9354 00140840 6

Library of Congress Cataloging-in-Publication Data

Askari, Fred K.
    Hepatitis C, the silent epidemic : the authoritative guide / Fred
K. Askari ; illustrations by Daniel S. Cutler.
        p.   cm.
    Includes bibliographical references and index.
    ISBN 0-306-46012-2
    1. Hepatits C--Popular works.   I. Title.
    [DNLM: 1. Hepatitis C.   WC 536 A834h 1999]
    RC848.H425A85   1999
    616.3'623--dc21
    DNLM/DLC
    for Library of Congress   99-11312
                                                                    CIP

This book is intended to provide a broad overview of hepatitis C infection and its many manifestations. Since hepatitis C can have wide-ranging effects which vary from individual to individual, specific disease management decisions can only be made by a patient in consultation with an examining physician. People should use this book as an adjunct to help from a liver specialist to answer their specific questions about hepatitis C. The practice of medicine is an art and may vary from one physician to the next; statements in this book should not be taken as dogma as some areas of knowledge remain controversial. Individuals infected with hepatitis C should remain in touch with a liver specialist and keep their care up to date. Dr. Bates and the patient characters in the book are fictitious, resemblence to any real people is a coincidence. CAUTION: List of drug side-effects and uses is not meant to be complete. Consult a physician, pharmacist, and appropriate references for more detailed complete information.

ISBN 0-306-46012-2

© 1999 Fred K. Askari
Kluwer Academic / Plenum Publishers
233 Spring Street, New York, N.Y. 10013

10 9 8 7 6 5 4 3 2 1

A C.I.P. record for this book is available from the Library of Congress

All rights reserved

No part of this book may be reproduced, stored in a retrieval system, or transmitted in any form or by any means, electronic, mechanical, photocopying, microfilming, recording, or otherwise, without written permission from the Publisher

Printed in the United States of America

To the tens of millions of people
who suffer with hepatitis C infection throughout the world

Contents

Preface

Back in the early 1980s, people started getting violently ill and dying from a new disease then known as gay-related immune deficiency syndrome, or GRID. Eventually we came to know this illness as AIDS, and scientists in France and America take credit for discovering its cause, the virus formally known as HIV. HIV, like other viruses, is a microscopic composition of protein and nucleic acid molecules. What is particularly perplexing about this virus is that the initial infection is often not noticed, and the deadly consequences of chronic infection are often not felt until years after the initial infection occurred.

As a student studying medicine at the time of onset of the HIV epidemic, I was struck by the vast array of diseases with unknown causes. One intriguing question is whether, given that HIV can infect someone and pass undetected only to manifest as disease many years later, there are other viruses that infect the body and cause injury years or decades later. Could cancer or liver disease be an endpoint of a chronic infection just like AIDS?

The answers to these questions are coming into sharper focus only recently. What is now known is that many cases of liver disease and liver cancer can be attributed to chronic viral infection. In 1989, a second virus which causes persistent infection—hepatitis C, or *HCV*—was identified. Hepatitis C causes one-third of all cases of chronic hepatitis leading to cirrhosis, liver failure, and liver cancer. Most of these cases were previously called "cryptogenic," which means we did not know what caused them. Now medical researchers have identified the cause of most cases of cryptogenic cirrhosis as a chronic viral infection, hepatitis C, which has been infecting the human population for decades. Like HIV, hepatitis C infection generally results in a chronic persistent infection with signs of disease often showing up years or decades after the initial infection. What is striking about hepatitis C, in contrast to HIV, is that about 2% of the United States population was already infected with hepatitis C when the virus was first discovered. HIV is 4-fold less common.

One of the challenges delaying the discovery of hepatitis C is that people infected with this virus come to medical attention for many different reasons. Hepatitis C is a master of disguise and intrigue, like an actor who can wear many different costumes and play a repertoire of characters. The appearance of the disease can be quite variable from person to person. The signs of hepatitis C infection that bring individuals to the attention of a physician may take many different forms. Abnormal blood tests can be discovered on routine screening. Infected individuals may have symptoms of tiredness or chronic fatigue. They may be plagued with joint aches, a rash, hives, or kidney problems. Finally, in more advanced cases, hepatitis C–infected people may suffer from liver failure. Once the liver becomes scarred over in the patient with hepatitis C infection, liver cancer occurs at a rate of 1–2% per year. Liver cancer is frightening because the treatments for most cases of liver cancer are not very effective.

This virus poses an immense problem. Hepatitis C persistently infects approximately 2% of the United States population, which translates into over 4 million people. The best estimates are that of those 4 million, approximately 20%—800,000 Americans—will progress to cirrhosis, liver failure, or liver cancer at some point in their lives. Hepatitis C is the leading necessitator of liver transplantation in the United States. Hepatitis C therefore poses a major public health risk. It is also a substantial cause of anxiety for those who are diagnosed, many of whom have chronic or ongoing symptoms such as fatigue and joint soreness.

Thousands of people are being told daily that they are infected with this virus. They want more answers than they can get from a simple pamphlet readily available at a physician's office or from a brief encounter with a physician. The concerns extend to other individuals such as spouses, sexual partners, coworkers, and other family members. The hepatitis C virus is such a pernicious and growing health problem that everyone needs to learn about it.

The huge pool of chronically infected people have many questions about the virus and few good answers. It is my aim to make readily available the truth about hepatitis C: how the virus was discovered, whom it infects, current treatments, emerging future treatments, and important precautions to prevent infection. Much of this information has only recently become available, and a large part of even the medical population is still poorly educated with regard to this virus. Through relating experiences of people with this dreadful infection, I hope to put a human face on this disease so that the reader may come to appreciate the impact of infection and understand its various symptoms and outcomes.

1

The Illness

Dr. Robert Bates was relieved to be finishing his internal medicine residency in 1989, having spent a great deal of effort learning to be a physician. He enjoyed helping people, but the grind of his day-to-day routine eventually grew tiresome. After 4 years in medical school studying facts and learning what caused some diseases, he had spent 3 years in his residency program learning more practical issues of daily patient care. He was delighted that this chapter in his training was coming to a close.

As an intern, one did not have much time to think about long-term problems or get to know patients over a significant period of time. Bates' job was to react to immediate problems—in essence to put out fires. Once he had heard a senior surgical house officer scold one of his young colleagues, "Neal, if you feel yourself starting to think, pick up the phone and page someone." Dr. Bates was looking forward to being able to think about the diseases that lacked good treatments and study new cures for some of these diseases so that he could better serve his patients, rather than just treat their symptoms. He wanted more than a band-aid approach to medicine.

At that moment, a nurse paged him to 5-West, because a patient had just become seriously short of breath. Dr. Bates hurried to see what was happening; he thought it could be quite critical and that time was of the essence. He quickly ticked off in his mind what might be wrong as he rushed down the corridor. Five West always had a distinctive odor, an institutional disinfectant that had been quite common in the 1950s but which had since fallen out of favor for more contemporary, more pleasant aromas. He could anticipate his arrival before he turned the corner and veered down the corridor as the smell of 5-West filled his nostrils. When he arrived, there was a patient, a veteran soldier, breathing 20 or 30 times a minute, perched on his bed like a pregnant Buddha. He was struggling to move air in and out of his lungs—something most of us take for granted. One could see at a glance the patient's belly bulging outward and upward under his hospital gown. It was so big that it got in the way of his lungs as he breathed.

"You gotta tap me, Doc," Rudy uttered between gasps. "I need to have some of this fluid drained off tonight." This once-strong man, a former Marine, now had thin and wasted muscles on the sides of his head. His forearms were thin with loose, floppy skin. He was gaunt and emaciated except for his ankles, which were swollen with fluid, only emphasizing how weak and helpless he looked altogether. "Whenever I get like this I need some of the fluid drawn off so I can breathe better. I need it done tonight," he plaintively said.

"Not a problem," Bates uttered. "I'll be back in a minute." He knew it was a problem in the long term, but things would probably be all right tonight. On this night, in this smelly hospital ward, the prognosis for the next several hours loomed heavily and was all that seemed to matter to Rudy and Dr. Bates. Dr. Bates hurried to get the angiocatheter, tubing, and vacuum lines to perform a paracentesis to drain the ascites from the patient's abdomen. He also got an Informed Consent sheet. When he returned to the room, he started to explain the procedure to Rudy.

Anguished, Rudy said, "Yeah, yeah, I've heard it all before. You clean off my side, you numb it with some medicine, then you stick the needle into my belly and drain off the fluid. If something goes wrong, it can get infected or there can be bleeding." He grabbed the paper and signed it in mock disgust at the delay in delivering comfort to him.

The clear yellow fluid flowed out of his belly through the tube into a vacuum bottle. As they drained it off, Rudy told Dr. Bates his story. "I once lost 60 pounds," he said. "You know, I was a POW in Vietnam. My platoon was moving quickly, and they lost me in the jungle. I had to walk for 3 days without food. Then I got to some river and yelled at some GIs on the other side; they turned out to be North Vietnamese. I was so messed up I thought they were some of us. They came in a boat and got me; I spent 4 years in prison—you know, the Hanoi Hilton. When the war ended I came home. I was fine for 25 years, then a couple of years ago I started swelling up."

"So, what do they think caused your liver to fail?" Bates asked.

"I don't know," Rudy said. "They don't know either. I drink a couple of beers now and then but no more than the next guy. They checked me for hepatitis A and B but I never got those. My liver enzymes have been slightly elevated for years." The doctor had a keen sense for the obvious—a scar on Rudy's arm above a tattoo that read "Mom."

"You were wounded in the war, weren't you? Did you get any blood transfusions then?" Bates stammered. "Yeah, I got a couple of pints of blood to top off my tank," Rudy said.

Dr. Bates put his arm on Rudy's shoulder. Rudy trembled for several seconds then started to breathe easier. Six or 7 liters of fluid had been taken off, and he was feeling more comfortable now. The doctor removed the catheter and covered the area with a bandage.

Rudy was like many other people in the late 1980s. He had cirrhosis, or scarring over, of the liver, but no one knew what caused it. He had a tattoo and a history of blood transfusions, both risk factors for transmission of viral hepatitis. But none of the tests available at the time could detect any of the known hepatitis viruses which might have caused Rudy's problem. Rudy had a tiny virus living in his liver. It is incredible to think that a tiny particle invisible to the eye and to even the most advanced microscopes of Rudy's youth had been living in him for some 30 years. He had been feeling okay until only recently. Now, the symptoms of decompensated cirrhosis had set in, in particular the accumulation of fluid in his belly (ascites).

Later we would learn that Rudy and millions of people like him had been infected with hepatitis C. This virus had lived within their livers for decades, sometimes causing symptoms early on, but frequently, as in Rudy's case, not making themselves evident until many years after infection. Now, however, the virus was taking its toll. Rudy's liver was scarred over. While some of his symptoms of cirrhosis might be controlled, at this stage nothing short of transplantation would restore Rudy's vigor.

Hepatitis C has many symptomatic profiles. The virus can manifest itself in many different ways, giving its victims any number of symptoms. Early symptoms can be limited to fatigue. The incubation period can also be extremely variable; people may be infected for decades before they experience any symptoms at all. There are reports of people infected with hepatitis C who have led normal lives for 50 or 60 years only to develop liver tumors later in life. Some people infected with hepatitis C may never develop symptoms and ultimately fall to an unrelated disease. In contrast, some people who were infected only briefly have progressed to liver failure. In addition, because of a symptom-free period which can last as long as 6 decades, studies to address the outcome of hepatitis C infection have been difficult to perform. As the disease progresses, symptoms of hepatitis C infection can include muscle aches, fatigue, a yellow skin color, abdominal pain, weakness, fluid retention, confusion, easy bruisability, and bleeding. Not everyone experiences all or any of these symptoms. Quite a bit about the biology and prognosis of people infected with hepatitis C is known, and the hardest part in communicating this information is the great variability from individual to individual.

Since the time the virus was discovered in 1989, much promising work has been done to develop effective treatments.

First, there are strategies to eradicate or get rid of the virus. These include injecting molecules that will stimulate the infected person's own immune system to attack the virus, as well as drugs that directly inhibit the virus from replicating or functioning. There also has been extensive experience with herbal and other home remedies.

Michael Houghton and his research team discovered the hepatitis C virus in 1989; following the filing of appropriate patents, the discovery was publicized. Excellent diagnostic tests to thoroughly screen all blood products prior to transfusion were not available until 1992. Therefore anyone who received a blood transfusion or blood products prior to 1992 is still at risk for having contracted hepatitis C. The enormity of this risk to the general population is staggering. Fully over 90% of transfusion-related hepatitis was caused by hepatitis C. The need to screen blood and blood products donated for transfusion approaches 50–70 million units of blood worldwide annually. At present, the blood supply in the United States is quite safe, but this is not true in all areas of the world. Certainly if one requires medical care in some areas of the third world, the risk of acquiring hepatitis C or even HIV may be significant. Future efforts to ensure the safety of the blood supply throughout the world clearly warrant support as a public health concern.

The ravaging symptoms of this disease make us all the more appreciative of the beauty of a functioning liver. The liver has several important functions, and we each need a functioning liver to live. The liver constitutes 12% of the human body and can be viewed as a bustling factory which makes important regulatory and housekeeping proteins. Simultaneously, the liver is hard at work metabolizing or modifying no-longer-needed proteins or foreign molecules, such as drugs, so the body may rid itself of them. As part of its maintenance role, it is one of the primary energy stores for the body, responding to fluctuating insulin levels to build or break down large sugar molecules. This explains in part why people with liver disease may have difficulty regulating their blood sugars

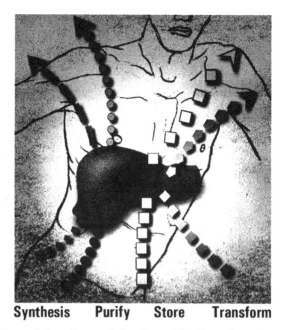

Synthesis   Purify   Store   Transform

Figure 1. Normal functions of the liver. The liver functions to make or synthesize proteins, purify or breakdown wastes, store carbohydrates and release them as an energy source, and metabolize or transform things like alcohol and many drugs. One cannot live without a functioning liver.

and may be fatigued. The liver makes clotting factors, proteins that circulate in the blood allowing it to clot when the skin is cut. This is one of several reasons that people with liver disease have bleeding tendencies.

What can cause hepatitis or inflammation of the liver besides hepatitis C? There are four other common viruses as well as several fairly common medical conditions that can lead to hepatitis. Hepatitis C must be differentiated from those conditions. Unfortunately, having one disease does not make one immune to another, so hepatitis C infection can coexist with these other conditions. Naturally, having two or more insulting injuries to the liver simultaneously carries with it a worse prospect than if only one problem exists.

VIRUSES THAT CAUSE HEPATITIS

Hepatitis A is transmitted primarily by an oral–fecal route. This is the hepatitis virus that is most commonly transmitted through imported fruits and vegetables. Field workers in a foreign country may not have access to a toilet as they pick strawberries or raspberries, and may defecate in the field during the course of their daily work. Human feces then contaminates the strawberries, which are subsequently shipped to the United States. In one such instance, schoolchildren in Michigan were exposed to the hepatitis A virus by eating strawberries supplied by a foreign food processor. Obviously this is a somewhat unpleasant prospect, but it is important to note that hepatitis A infection is usually self-limiting, meaning that it goes away on its own, and while people may be quite sick at the time, long-term consequences of hepatitis A infection are less common.

In contrast, hepatitis B infection can generally lead to three different potential outcomes. The infection may be acute but still cleared by an immune response from the body, leading to a resistance to subsequent infection. Another possibility is an acute phase followed by a chronic phase in which the immune response is not adequate to clear the viral infection, leaving a chronic form of infection, much like can occur with hepatitis C. In the worst case the infection passes to a fulminant phase in which the liver actually fails and the person either gets a liver transplant or dies. This occurs only with about 2–3% of hepatitis B infections, but obviously merits attention nevertheless.

About 15% of hepatitis C infections resolve within weeks of infection and do not progress to a chronic, persistent viral hepatitis. This small fraction of hepatitis C infections are termed cases of acute hepatitis. People who have had acute hepatitis C, however, are not necessarily immune to subsequent challenges from the virus. The vast majority of cases of hepatitis C infection do go on to chronic hepatitis C infection.

Hepatitis C is therefore the agent that is most commonly responsible for chronic viral hepatitis in this country.

Hepatitis D, or delta virus, is a hitchhiker, entering cells by binding to a piece of hepatitis B, the surface antigen protein, and therefore hepatitis D infects only people who either are actively infected with hepatitis B or are chronic carriers of hepatitis B. It is rather like a parasite. It also leads to persistent infection or chronic infection and is more common in people who have acquired their hepatitis B infection through intravenous drug use rather than other routes, such as sexual intercourse or blood transfusion. Hepatitis B is much easier to catch through sexual intercourse than either HIV or HCV. Hepatitis C is relatively difficult to catch through sexual intercourse in comparison with either of those other two viruses, although sexual transmission of hepatitis C is still possible.

Hepatitis E is another viral cause of liver inflammation that is more common in the developing world than in the United States. This hepatitis virus is also transmitted predominantly by ingesting feces tainted with hepatitis E. Most cases consist of an acute hepatitis from which people recover fully. One unusual aspect of hepatitis E virus infection is that the disease runs a much more aggressive course in pregnant women, with up to 20% dying from the infection. Hepatitis E is very rare in the United States and is responsible primarily for an acute form of hepatitis in travelers returning from endemic areas such as Africa.

There are good vaccines available for hepatitis A and for hepatitis B, and hepatitis D is indirectly prevented by vaccination against its obligate coinfection, hepatitis B. These should be given to all people who have known liver disease and to people who travel to areas where those viruses are endemic, such as the Caribbean. Youngsters in the United States are being immunized with the hepatitis B vaccine, after the dismal failure of an effort to immunize focus groups such as homosexual men, healthcare workers, and intravenous drug users. The vaccine is safe. Since it only contains a piece of the hepatitis B virus, no one can contract the infection by being vaccinated. The vaccine appears to provide protection through immunologic memory for at least several decades and perhaps a lifetime.

It should be noted that the liver is sometimes infected by other viruses, albeit rarely. These include Epstein-Barr virus (EBV), cytomegalovirus (CMV), herpes simplex virus (HSV), and adenovirus (Ad). Some of these infections tend more frequently to infect the livers of immunocompromised people, such as those infected with HIV or suffering from cancer.

NONVIRAL CAUSES OF HEPATITIS

Hepatitis or inflammation of the liver can also be caused by things other than viruses. One cause is autoimmune hepatitis, in which the person's own immune system attacks the liver, leading to inflammation and hepatocellular necrosis. What causes a body to turn on itself and use the weapons designed to protect it from outside invaders to destroy itself? That is a very good question and is the subject of active research. Another cause of liver inflammation is Wilson's disease, an inherited genetic defect in the body's ability to handle copper properly. In this disease the copper accumulates in the liver, causing inflammation. Other symptoms associated with Wilson's disease include neurologic deterioration and copper-colored circles inside the eyes. Another inherited cause of liver disease is hemochromatosis, a genetic defect in the ability to regulate iron absorption and accumulation in the liver and in other organs. The depositing of iron in the liver can lead to inflammation and ultimately fibrotic scarring or cirrhosis of the liver. This is one of the more common genetic defects, affecting up to 1% of Caucasian people of European descent. The carrier state for this condition, heterozygous hemochromatosis, has been associated with increased fibrosis in hepatitis C-infected individuals as well.

Another cause of liver inflammation is α-1 antitrypsin deficiency (α-1 AT deficiency). α-1 AT is a circulating protein made

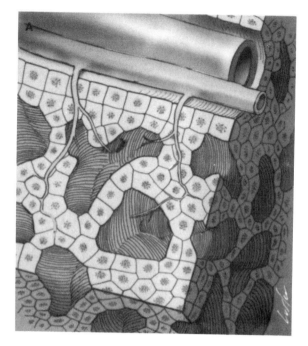

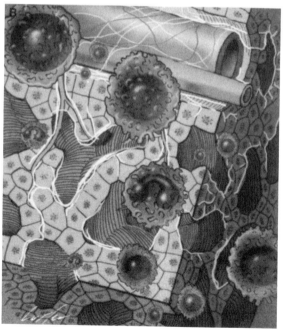

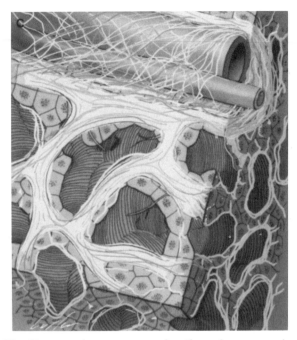

Figure 2. The liver, as it appears under the microscope, in health and disease. Panel A shows the appearance of the normal liver cells without inflammation, fibrosis, or scar tissue. Besides the liver cells, the illustration shows a branch of a portal vein, which delivers blood to the liver, and a branch of a bile duct, which drains fluids from the liver into the bowel. Panel B shows the liver with a response to hepatitis C infection: inflammation as represented by lurking immune cells hovering into the liver to fight the invading virus and increased fibrosis or scar tissue (white lines). Panel C shows the liver with more advanced fibrosis (scarring) leading to cirrhosis. Note that the inflammatory activity or immune cells infiltrating the liver may actually decrease once cirrhosis has occurred.

in the liver. α-1 AT functions to inhibit elastase, a protein which breaks down other molecules into tiny snippets. Elastase is used to protect the body from foreign attack. When it is not properly regulated by α-1 AT, elastase can break down important structural molecules in the lung. Liver toxicity occurs in about 20% of people with α-1 AT deficiency. The mechanism of this injury is unique, resulting from the buildup of misfolded, defective protein in the liver. This leads to inflammation in the liver and can lead to scarring or fibrosis.

Other forms of hepatitis or inflammation of the liver may result from adverse drug reactions, drug toxicities or toxic reactions to herbs or chemicals. The most common hepato-inflammatory agent of this type is alcohol. Alcohol is broken down in the liver. An individual who drinks too much alcohol can develop inflammation in the liver and eventually deposition of fat and scar tissue in the liver. All of these forms of liver toxicity may coexist with hepatitis C infection, and when they do their combined injury is often more than would be anticipated from the simple additive toxicities. Hepatitis C can cause synergistic injury with other liver toxins; this effect is best appreciated with alcohol.

THE COURSE OF INFECTION

Symptoms of liver damage, such as fatigue or flulike symptoms, usually are not felt by infected people until the hepatitis C virus has spread throughout the liver, which can take 6 weeks. Frequently, the period of initial or acute infection with hepatitis C passes unnoticed, and chronic infection may be present for decades prior to the diagnosis of hepatitis C infection. Importantly, there are usually enough viral particles in the serum 2 weeks after infection to spread the disease to another person should blood-to-blood contact occur. Hepatitis C is characterized by a dangerous, symptomless infectious period which may last for decades. During this period, the liver may be damaged beyond repair, and the virus may be unwittingly transmitted to other people.

Why does the immune system, which is so facile at clearing so many other viral infections, fail to clear hepatitis C in about 85% of cases of infection? One answer is that hepatitis C has evolved to be too good at its job at attacking the body and setting up shop inside of liver cells. Many new therapies for

Table 1.   Hepatitis C at a Glance

35,000–40,000 new infections every year, the majority of which are symptom free

85% of infected individuals fail to fight off the virus naturally and 70% of infected individuals progress to chronic disease

4 million people chronically infected in the U.S.

2% of the U.S. population is infected with hepatitis C

50% of chronic liver disease is caused by hepatitis C

At least 20% of hepatitis C-infected patients progress to cirrhosis within 20 years of infection

About one in four people with hepatitis C-induced cirrhosis will progress to liver failure

At least 10,000 U.S. deaths are attributable to hepatitis annually.

Tens of thousands of hospitalizations are necessary for hepatitis C annually

Thousands of liver transplants for hepatitis C-related liver failure annually in the U.S.

Nine out of 10 infected people are not aware of their diagnosis

hepatitis C are designed to boost the body's immune system and help it fight off the virus.

To summarize, hepatitis is inflammation of the liver. It has several potential causes, including viral infections, genetic diseases, and direct chemical or drug toxicities. There are really only four primary types of viral hepatitis which are common in the United States: hepatitis A, hepatitis B, hepatitis C, and hepatitis D. The existence of more than one viral infection at a time does occur. Careful consideration of multiple potential causes of liver inflammation is warranted in people found to be infected with hepatitis C. By far the most common cause of chronic hepatitis is hepatitis C.

There are many diseases that may cause hepatitis. The disease that causes the majority of cases of chronic hepatitis is a virus called hepatitis C. The viral infection takes different courses in different people, with the rate of progression to cirrhosis or scarring over of the liver ranging from years to decades. Often, infected people experience a prolonged symptom-free period of infection during which they may transmit the disease to their friends, family, and strangers if simple precautions are not followed. The disease may cause fatigue, aches, and pains, and hepatitis C is an emerging public health problem. It is getting strong attention because of the dramatic effects of hepatitis C-induced liver failure now being experienced by a fraction of infected people. While the disease has existed for decades, the virus that causes it was only recently discovered. We are only recently learning how best to diagnose, treat, and manage hepatitis C infection.

2

Discovering
Hepatitis C

For decades, people suffered with end-stage liver disease labeled "cryptogenic" cirrhosis, which simply meant we did not know what had caused the liver disease. Some people who received blood transfusions and then developed hepatitis were diagnosed with non-A, non-B hepatitis or transfusion-associated hepatitis. The story of how hepatitis C, the agent that caused most cases of cryptogenic cirrhosis and non-A, non-B viral hepatitis, was discovered is uplifting, as it is a testament to the inquisitive and persistent human nature to fight disease.

Discovering the cause of many cases of cirrhosis was an area of pressing research focus for many years. It had long been known that blood transfusions were associated with many cases of hepatitis. Before 1989, every blood transfusion carried with it an appreciable risk—as high as 10%—of transmitting hepatitis or inflammation of the liver.

The main thing hepatitis A, B, and C share is that they are all viruses that infect the liver; these viruses also differ in many ways. Initially, tests were developed for hepatitis B, which replicates in the liver to very high levels and secretes very high quantities of viral proteins. These viral proteins stimulate a robust immune response, and circulating antibodies to components of hepatitis B were easy to detect. Furthermore, the virus can quite easily be visualized by electron microscopy. Hepatitis B was the first source of hepatitis acquired through donors' blood that began to be screened. The donated units of blood were screened for the presence of hepatitis B antibodies and snippets of virus called surface antigens, in other words any units containing evidence of hepatitis B.

Hepatitis A was also relatively easy to screen for, and blood from people with this condition was not used for transfusion as tests for hepatitis A were developed. Therefore, the remaining cases of hepatitis from transfusion were termed non-A, non-B hepatitis. It was relatively easy to identify some cases of hepatitis which came from units of blood that contained the transmissible agent for non-A, non-B hepatitis; the hepatitis would set in weeks after a transfusion. Before the discovery of hepatitis C, however, it was not known whether there was predominantly one agent or if there were many different agents which conferred this mysterious hepatitis. As we now know, only one virus, hepatitis C, makes up the vast majority of what used to be termed non-A, non-B hepatitis.

The cause of non-A, non-B hepatitis was elusive because the hepatitis C virus does not stimulate as strong an immune response as, for example, the hepatitis B virus, which made screening for hepatitis C very difficult. Eventually, scientists were able to isolate the hepatitis C virus through a relatively straightforward technique. They were actually able to use a unit of blood to transmit hepatitis C from a human donor to a chimpanzee. They used this infectious serum, which they were pretty certain contained a virus that caused hepatitis, to discover hepatitis C. They took the serum and isolated the RNA, which contains instructions for how to make proteins. They then used this RNA to make actual viral proteins inside of cells. In this technique, the RNA from the serum is placed into cells in tissue culture incubators in a laboratory. In other words, the RNA is then decoded in the cells to make viral proteins. The RNA is like a computer program that contains the code or instructions for making hepatitis C virus particles as well as other proteins. In this way, the viral RNA causes the manufacture of viral proteins in these tissue culture cells along with other proteins.

The next challenge is to isolate the cells that are expressing the hepatitis C proteins. This is a bit like hunting for a needle in a haystack, but fortunately they had serum which contained antibodies to the hepatitis C proteins. The antibodies are like a magnet which specifically binds to the needle as one sifts through the hay. This makes the job easier. So once they had the cells, some of which made the hepatitis C virus pieces, the cells were searched with serum that contains antibodies to viral proteins. Some of the cells in culture will contain viral RNA and express viral protein. By using patient serum containing antibodies to the infectious agent one can screen and identify the cells that react with the serum antibodies against hepatitis C. These cells contain the viral protein, allowing investigators to isolate portions of the viral agent hepatitis C. Chiron researchers patented the virus soon after isolating it.

This 1989 discovery was very exciting and led to successful efforts to develop diagnostic tests for hepatitis C. The most urgent priority, of course, was to screen the blood supply. We are now able to ensure the safety of our blood supply by excluding units of blood that contain antibodies to hepatitis C. Researchers did this by taking the snippets of isolated hepatitis C RNA and making hepatitis C proteins for use in diagnostic tests to figure out which units of blood were safe to transfuse into other people. Similar tests are used to figure out who is infected with hepatitis C.

The discovery of hepatitis C was an important step forward in fighting hepatitis C's debilitating symptoms. Indeed, discovery of the virus allowed us to begin to understand the magnitude of the public health problem hepatitis C defines. Michael Houghton and his colleagues at Chiron Corporation discovered the disease-causing agent in 1989. The company has its headquarters outside of San Francisco in Emeryville, CA, at the foot of the Bay Bridge. As a result of this significant discovery, Chiron's stock value shot up. Since that initial enthusiasm, investor interest has plateaued somewhat since the translation of the discovery of the virus to products other than diagnostic tests has occurred at a slower pace than initially anticipated. This reflects the difficult time the entire pharmaceutical industry has had developing effective treatments and vaccines for hepatitis C.

Of interest to people infected with hepatitis C, Chiron has active research programs in antiviral therapy as well as in vaccines for hepatitis C. They are currently conducting a hepatitis C vaccine trial sanctioned by the FDA. Chiron has a number of strong competitors in these areas of research, and the potential success of any of these drugs is speculative.

One area of emerging hepatitis C research is the development of drugs which function as antiviral therapies. Because the virus grows inside cells, many of the traditional approaches to developing drugs would not apply. Many classical drugs bind to the surface of cells such as calcium channel blockers, antihypertensives known as beta blockers and other commonly used medicines. To treat an intracellular virus, the drug must cross the cell membrane to enter the cell and interact with the virus. For this reason, molecules called "small molecules" in the pharmaceutical industry are being studied to interact with the hepatitis C virus because they penetrate to the inside of cells more easily than do larger molecules. One successful example of small-molecule drugs includes the extremely successful protease inhibitors that have revolutionized treatments for HIV. Similar strategies are being tested for interaction to develop small-molecule therapies for hepatitis C.

The hepatitis C virus is composed of a single strand of RNA viral nucleic acids attached to a core protein and surrounded by an envelope of viral proteins. It is like the Trojan horse the Greeks left outside the gates of Troy as if it were a gift. The Trojans brought it inside the city walls, allowing the craftily disguised soldiers inside to accomplish what thousands of attacking soldiers had failed to do: penetrate the fortress walls of the city of Troy. Once inside, the first soldier quietly slid out of the horse using weapons he snuck in with him to open city gates, enabling more Greek attackers to ransack the city. One can envision the envelope proteins functioning much like the mythic horse. The virus' coat uses trickery to evade the immune system (city defenders) and enter the cell. Once inside the cell, the virus replicates itself over and over again, allowing more attackers to ransack the cell. The trickery the virus uses to get inside the cells is to constantly change its appearance so that the virus may subvert the body's immune system, which tries to protect the cells from invasion.

This variation in hepatitis C is reflected by many viral genotypes or strains of the virus which exist throughout the world. These genotypes reflect the classification of different hepatitis C infections from one individual to another based on the similarities or differences in their genetic makeup, much as Europeans of Swedish descent are more similar to other Swedes than to Germans, for example. Some genotypes are more common in some areas of the world than others, reflecting transmission patterns. At present, genotypes are checked as part of some experimental protocols to try to learn more about how the hepatitis C virus changes. Some studies have revealed differences in the way hepatitis C virus infections classified in different genotypes respond to interferon. Some genotypes have been correlated with an improved probability of response to interferon. It is not clear why some hepatitis C genotypes have a more favorable response rate than do others. It may just be, for example, that people infected with a certain genotype have a shorter average duration of infection than do those infected with another genotype. We do not routinely check hepatitis C genotypes of every infected individual unless they are on a study protocol, as this information is not generally used in managing an individual's treatment.

Within an infected individual, there are many quasi-species or different strains of the virus which reflect the constant changing appearance of the virus to avoid the immune system. These changes make it extremely difficult for the immune system to respond effectively to the infection; in essence, it must respond to a broad range of different virus appearances which are constantly changing. New approaches to treatment with drugs that augment the immune system are used, but there is still a long way to go in improving them. New types of drugs are also being developed to attack the virus directly.

Drug companies are working to develop new drugs to treat hepatitis C. One approach is to develop compounds similar to those used to fight HIV, the virus that causes AIDS. It is important to recognize, though, that none of the new approaches to HIV treatment thus far lead to elimination of the HIV viral infection from the body. In present studies, they simply decrease the amount of HIV virus in the body and prolong the course of the infection. That is one reason why our having interferon, which can cure hepatitis C infection (albeit in only a small fraction of the number of infected patients), is so remarkable.

One note of caution about the drugs under development is that there is a fair amount of variability in the structure from one strain of hepatitis C to another. Therefore, resistance to any virus inhibitor that becomes available may be a concern. In the case of HIV, it has been found that resistance does develop to the inhibitors over time, and cocktails of two or three or even four inhibitors at once may be used to treat HIV in order to prevent or overcome the development of resistant viral strains. It is therefore believed that multiple hepatitis C inhibitors will be developed, but they may not be active against all forms of hepatitis C, and resistance may develop to these molecules over time. It is hoped that between combinations of interferon and virus inhibitors a greater percentage of infected people may be cured of their hepatitis C viral infection.

THE MEDICAL COMMUNITY'S RESPONSE

Dr. Bates had heard the buzz in the liver community. The National Institutes of Health consensus conference on hepatitis C was going to be big, and there were ads in all of the professional journals inviting everyone to attend. Bates got his invitation in the mail. All of the big players in the field would be there. He drove to Washington and checked in at the Bethesda Holiday Inn. In the morning the hotel shuttle was jammed with conference attendees, so Bates made the 10-minute walk through the parklike National Institutes of Health campus to the Natcher Building conference room.

Held in March of 1997, the goal of the conference was quite simple: to wade through the evidence about hepatitis C's actions and generate a concise summary of our current state of knowledge. One problem with developing a consensus in this or any field is that individuals working in the area of hepatitis C research have a vested interest in propelling their own ideas to the forefront and having others accept their theories. This leads to a healthy climate of debate within a given scientific or clinical field, but can also be rather confusing for both experts and general practitioners who need succinct information to manage the daily practices of their patients. The concept of the consensus conference was to bring together a panel of individuals who are knowledgeable judges but not vested in the field of hepatitis C research. This panel included the clergy, business people, ethicsts and some medical doctors. The conference was headed by a distinguished gastroenterologist, Dr. Don Powell, who was admired for his knowledge about liver diseases while having no direct involvement in hepatitis C research, and thus unbiased.

The members of the committee received a tall order: to sift through the often ambiguous literature, read and hear the testimony of experts in the field and generate a concise, lucid statement on the current state of affairs in the field of hepatitis C research and care. The panel had received documents to review several weeks prior to the meeting, and then heard the presentations of about two dozen expert "witnesses" over several days. Following the presentations, there were several periods set aside for questions, comments and debate. The presentations occurred in a public conference room at the National

Institutes of Health, and anyone in the field (or even the public) who wished could attend the conference. This was not the kind of closed-door elitist meeting that Bates had become so accustomed to attending. Rather, over 2000 people attended it. Next, the panel of 12 adjourned to a meeting room and in a remarkable overnight feat wrote the consensus statement, which consisted of a brief pamphlet outlining their perceptions of the facts relating to hepatitis C research and clinical care. This draft was then copied and distributed to the general participants in the conference for public discussion.

Based on the critique discussed, a final "consensus statement" was subsequently prepared. Certainly all of the members of the panel, let alone the 2000 people attending the conference, did not agree on every point. However, the conference did generate a valid summary of the then current knowledge of hepatitis C, and this summary has served as a springboard for future investigation and clinical action to further the care of patients suffering with hepatitis C.

Many of the conclusions reached in the consensus statements remain valid today, but a great deal of change has occurred in our knowledge of hepatitis C in the year and a half subsequent to the conference. Bates reflected that the greatest legacy of the consensus conference will no doubt be that it thrust the issue of hepatitis C infection into the forefront of public consciousness. It was once fashionable in the medical community to deny the importance of hepatitis C infection. Following the conference, there was no longer a state of denial toward the long-term ramifications of hepatitis C infection and the utility of currently available therapy. The public was also first made aware of the potential danger lurking within the livers of so many unsuspecting Americans by the publicity the conference generated. Bates drove home happy that he had participated, and excited more than ever to tackle head-on the problems of his nemesis.

For the first time, there was a clear set of guidelines which stated that patients eligible for interferon treatment should receive it. Risk factors for transmission of this bloodborne

Table 2. Key Points of Future Hepatitis C Research
___
Obtain more information about transmission
Better understand why some people progress to cirrhosis faster than others
How should we screen for liver cancer?
How do people recover from hepatitis C infection?
How does the virus damage the liver?
Better understand how the virus functions on a molecular level
Better understand influence of alcohol use, obesity, diabetes mellitus, iron
    and other medications on disease progression
Develop more consistent and reliable tests for hepatitis C
Better understand costs of treatment and impact on quality of life
Develop a vaccine for hepatitis C
Better educate people about the disease; avoid transmission of the virus
___

virus were clearly discussed. Diagnostic tests were reviewed. Most important, the risk of just waiting to see what happened, denying that any action need be taken against hepatitis C, was clearly defined. Four out of five individuals with stable cirrhosis (scarring of the liver) would live over 10 years. In the absence of a liver transplant, one of two individuals with unstable cirrhosis (scarring complicated by fluid retention in the abdomen, bleeding from engorged stomach or food pipe veins, confusion, or muscle wasting) would live 5 more years. The need for vigorous efforts to fight hepatitis C and prevent its spread was clear.

3

Hepatitis C and Chronic Hepatitis

Hepatitis C generally infects a person silently. The individual may not even notice being sick, or he may later recall a flulike illness that corresponds with the time of infection. Nevertheless, it is not unusual for someone to learn of a hepatitis C infection decades after it occurs. Over 85% of people infected with hepatitis C develop a persistent, chronic infection. The high rate of chronic infection is one important difference between hepatitis C and hepatitis B. With hepatitis B the majority of people are able to clear their systems of the acute infection. With chronic hepatitis C, that's far less likely. As a matter of course, less than 15% of hepatitis C infections are cleared in the acute stage of infection. Moreover, the disease may be symptom-free or symptomatic. Those symptoms may include joint stiffness, muscle aches, sweats, nausea, vomiting, pains in the right side of the abdomen, or fatigue.

Other measures of viral infection that are used include measuring the levels of certain proteins called serum liver enzymes. As liver cells are injured or die, these proteins leak out into the bloodstream from hepatocytes (liver cells). There-fore, abnormal elevations of these proteins in the blood may reflect ongoing liver inflammation or damage. Unfortunately, during the course of hepatitis C infection, the levels of these enzymes fluctuate in the body. Therefore, isolated readings of these values are less useful than a series of measurements over time, which may provide a clearer picture of the severity of inflammation in the liver. One frequent mistake made by in-fected individuals and physicians is to rely too much upon the serum liver enzyme measurement. These serum liver enzymes can be used as markers, for example, in following treatment effectiveness and disease progression, but liver biopsy re-mains the gold standard for judging the severity of the disease. Some centers also use measurements of hepatitis C RNA in blood as another marker of infection. Finally, the immune response to infection may be measured by analyzing anti-bodies to hepatitis C in the blood.

TESTING FOR HEPATITIS C

Who is infected with hepatitis C? One urgency after dis-covering the virus was to determine which people were in-fected and to characterize the natural course of the disease. To determine which people were infected, screening tests were necessary. The first startling observation was that hepatitis C was predominantly associated with chronic forms of hepatitis. Though it is commonly symptomless at the time of infection, hepatitis C-infected individuals rarely can present with an acute hepatitislike picture. Next, the acute infection often turns into chronic inflammation in the liver. Therefore, a de-velopment of reliable tests for the virus was necessary. The first tests for evidence of viral infection involved tests for anti-bodies to hepatitis C virus. Later tests were more refined, assaying for antibodies toward more viral proteins—this to make sure that the screening tested positive for any person infected with the virus. A second goal was to improve the specificity of the tests, that is, to ensure that people who had a positive test were actually infected with the virus.

Judy is a 35-year-old mother of two who works in an ice cream store that provides a good disease prevention health-care plan. Judy, though without disease symptoms, went to see her doctor for a routine examination. She felt well, and although the physical examination revealed no causes for alarm, screening blood tests detected an elevation in her serum trans-aminases (liver enzymes). Further workup of her liver enzyme elevation revealed the presence of antibodies to the hepatitis C virus. Her initial reaction was one of disbelief. "How could I have gotten the virus?" she gasped. Judy had seen Rudy coming in her store for ice cream. Her impression of hepatitis C was that it was a severely debilitating disease. How could she have it too?

She did not have any of the common risk factors, which include blood transfusions prior to 1992, tattoos, history of intravenous drug use, hemodialysis, use of intranasal cocaine, or history of promiscuous sexual activity. *In up to 20% of people*, it is not possible to identify a clear source for the infection. To confirm that her antibodies actually reflected hepatitis C infection, a polymerase chain reaction (PCR) test was run and shown to be positive. The PCR tested for the presence of hepatitis C RNA in Judy's blood. Judy was horrified. "Why me?" she gasped. Then she told her doctor, "But I couldn't have liver disease; I never drink alcohol." Dr. Bates shuffled his feet and rubbed his eyes. He explained that anyone could catch hepatitis C, and that we really did not know why 20% of those found infected had contracted it.

Liver function tests refer to a standard laboratory measurement of liver health and function. These serum tests are run on samples of blood and are used throughout the country as an indirect measure of liver function and health. What the tests measure can be divided into four broad categories: (1) proteins produced by the liver which circulate and function throughout the body; (2) enzymes made within liver cells; (3) enzymes found predominantly in the cells of the biliary system which drains from the liver; and (4) breakdown products or molecules processed through the biliary system. The liver is a robust synthetic factory, so determination of the blood concentration of proteins commonly made in the liver is usually a good marker of liver function. The serum albumin and PT (prothrombin time) are generally measured to assess liver function. Albumin is a protein that circulates in high concentration in the blood and transports many molecules bound to it. It is an essential constituent of blood and helps to keep fluid within blood vessels rather than having it leak out into the extracellular space, which can lead to swollen ankles or intra-abdominal fluid collection, which is known as ascites.

The first test run on Judy's serum was to check for hepatitis C through the EIA test (enzyme-linked immunoassay), which is relatively sensitive but is not always as specific as some other tests for hepatitis C. Therefore it was necessary to confirm a positive EIA test through another test: the RIBA test, which stands for recombinant immunoblot assay, or hepatitis C PCR assay. The EIA and RIBA tests involved running actual reactions between the person's serum, which may or may not contain antibodies, and recombinant hepatitis C proteins. The RIBA test differs from the EIA test in that the blots are run with the virus proteins anchored to a special matrix, a fibrous support, which allows a more specific determination as to whether an EIA test is truly positive.

Finally, direct tests for viral RNA were developed. In general, a first- or second-generation EIA test is used for screening, and either a RIBA test or a hepatitis C RNA test is used for confirmation of the diagnosis. In patients with a high probability of hepatitis C infection based on exposure risk factors, sometimes the confirmatory tests may be foregone.

The use of PCR in clinical diagnostics has sparked a revolution in medicine. You may recall that the PCR test became famous during the O.J. Simpson trial; more recently, it was used to test a notorious blue dress for evidence of the president's semen.

Polymerase chain reaction tests started out as pure molecular biology in basic research labs and worked their way to clinical practice. This PCR test allows for the amplification of very small quantities of viral RNA to generate larger quantities of virus-derived DNA, which are easily detected on simple laboratory gels. Nevertheless, even this routine and simple test may have its difficulties. For example, if a serum sample is not properly processed and stored, the RNA may degrade. If the RNA degrades, then the reaction may not be as sensitive as it would have been if the samples had been properly processed. In the extreme situation, if a serum sample is quite old or has been stored incorrectly, the RNA may degrade completely and lead to the report of a false-negative RNA value. Similarly, because the RNA of the hepatitis C virus is highly variable, both from person to person and within one person, it is possible that the primers used to probe the patient's serum for the presence of hepatitis C viral RNA may not perfectly match every strain of virus. Primer mismatch also may lead to a false-negative test result.

More recently, efforts have been made to develop tests that quantify viral RNA. Viral RNA levels are reported as the number of particles of virus (virions) per milliliter (about 25 drops) of blood. While these measurements are intuitively attractive, they must be interpreted with several caveats. First, different labs may use different tests, some of which are still under development. Efforts are directed at trying to improve not only their accuracy in replicating reported quantities of viral particles in serially tested samples, but also their sensitivity—that is, their ability to detect smaller and smaller numbers of viral particles. Some of these tests have also come under a great deal of criticism because some labs do not run them properly. In a recent survey by the American College of Pathologists in which they mailed out samples of patients' serum containing known amounts of RNA, *up to 20% of the labs reported positive quantities of viral RNA when the patient's blood actually did not contain hepatitis C.* Naturally, this degree of variability from lab to lab is unacceptable, and there are growing measures being taken to regulate these molecular diagnostic labs more effectively so that these tests may be interpreted more reliably. In the interim, both people worried about their own infection and physicians treating these patients must interpret the hepatitis C RNA data they receive from some labs with cautious skepticism. It is important to recognize that the hepatitis C PCR assay is not licensed by the FDA in the United States for testing to determine who is infected with hepatitis C. While physicians order hepatitis C RNA tests routinely, results are often reported with the disclaimer, "for research use only." Greater efforts to improve the reliability of these tests are under way.

As measures of quantitative viral RNA become more reliable, these also may be useful in assessing disease progression. It should be noted that levels of viral RNA may fluctuate over time, just as the levels of serum liver enzymes may fluctuate over time. Therefore, a person holding his infection in relatively good check may all of a sudden see it break through, and viral RNA, as well as serum liver enzymes, may go up once again. It is provocative that this has been shown, at least in some people, to correlate with mutations or changes in the viral genome or RNA in areas which are vital to the body mounting an effective immune attack on the virus. These mutations are like a fugitive changing his clothes and putting on a fake moustache to slip away undetected. The mutations cause changes in the viral envelope or coating proteins which allow the virus to fight the body's immune system more effectively and proliferate more vigorously. Therefore, there is a need for both ongoing chronic monitoring, and ongoing recurrent physical examinations for people infected with hepatitis C.

Unfortunately, physicians fall short of curing an individual of hepatitis C infection in the majority of cases. For persistently infected individuals, hepatitis C needs to be treated like any other chronic medical condition such as diabetes or hypertension at its best, and at its worst, hepatitis C needs to be treated aggressively with even the potential for liver trans-

Table 3. Diagnostic Tests for Hepatitis C Infection

Antibody to the hepatitis C virus
  EIA (enzyme immunoassay) checks blood for antibodies; sensitive but not as specific as confirmatory RIBA test
  RIBA (recombinant immunoblot assay) more specific, often used to confirm a positive EIA
PCR (polymerase chain reaction) hepatitis C RNA assay
  Qualitative PCR hepatitis C RNA assay
  Quantitative PCR hepatitis C RNA assay
Branched chain quantitative hepatitis C RNA assay
Liver biopsy; confirms diagnosis with characteristic morphologic features correlating with infection

plantation. In between, there is a growing armory of therapies, both experimental and FDA approved, which may be used to treat people and eradicate the virus. The view is coming to prevail that anyone infected with the virus needs to be under the ongoing care of a physician knowledgeable in the rapid advances in hepatitis C treatment. Nevertheless, it is fair to say that the majority of people infected in this country with hepatitis C are not yet aware of their infection. Many physicians now advocate widespread screening of groups of people at high risk for infection. Naturally, this may be quite expensive, but it is also vital. For example, in random screenings of emergency room visitors at the Johns Hopkins Medical Center, up to 19% of the people coming to that inner-city emergency room were already infected with hepatitis C. In addition, epidemiologic studies have estimated that up to 10% of black males aged 40 to 50 may already be infected with hepatitis C.

There is a growing urgency to identify people at risk of spreading the infection further, as well as identifying those who need to be monitored and treated at this time. People who should be screened for hepatitis C are reviewed in Table 4. In addition, children born to mothers infected with hepatitis C should be tested at their 1-year checkup. Healthcare workers such as laboratory technicians, doctors, nurses and others involved in direct patient care who are exposed to hepatitis C containing blood by a needlestick, for example, should be tested. Finally, regular sexual partners of hepatitis C-infected people should be screened for the disease.

More medications to treat hepatitis C are becoming available. By not identifying infected individuals, the disease, like HIV, will only spread. For people who do not respond to the traditional treatments, there are a growing number of experimental therapies available at centers which perform clinical trials to assess efficacy of the new treatments. Referral to centers that have ongoing clinical trials for the treatment of hepatitis C seems to be prudent for the sufferer.

Before treatment, however, it is still necessary to confirm that hepatitis C is the sole source of the individual's liver inflammation. Since there are many liver diseases, the mere presence of hepatitis C infection does not make one immune to

Table 4. People Who Should Be Screened
for Hepatitis C Infection

People with a history of recreational intravenous drug use or snorting cocaine, regardless of when or how much they did

People who have received a letter from the Red Cross stating that they received blood from someone who was later determined to be hepatitis C infected

People on kidney hemodialysis

Anyone who received a blood transfusion before July 1992

Anyone who received an organ transplant like a liver, pancreas, heart, lungs, or kidney before July 1992

Anyone who received clotting factors derived from blood before 1987

Anyone who has shared razor blades

People with a history of multiple sexual partners, particularly if they caught another sexually transmitted disease such as syphilis, gonorrhea, or chlamydia

Anyone with HIV infection

Anyone exposed to blood in the healthcare field before the implementation of universal precautions

Anyone who has a tattoo

---

the other diseases. Therefore, the general approach to treating people with hepatitis C infection involves a liver biopsy prior to initiating treatment (with either an established and proven treatment regimen or an experimental protocol). Rarely, the hepatitis C infection may be so mild, that is there may be so little inflammation, that interferon treatment may be deferred. The biopsy is also necessary to exclude other forms of liver disease such as hemochromatosis, alpha-1 antitrypsin deficiency, Wilson's disease, autoimmune hepatitis or other forms of viral hepatitis. The liver biopsy is also necessary to see what stage the hepatitis C virus disease has reached. The liver biopsy is interpreted by a pathologist, who may confirm that the pattern of inflammation is consistent with hepatitis C infection or may suggest an alternative diagnosis. Many other conditions can cause inflammation in the liver, and frequently, as mentioned earlier, it is possible for a person to suffer from more than one condition. In the case of simultaneous multiple causes, one may be aware of and treat all potential etiologies in order to provide the individual infected with hepatitis C the best possible care. The liver biopsy is also used to tell how badly the liver is damaged and to estimate disease prognosis. The results of the liver biopsy guide treatment, too, and a very sick liver may be treated differently from a relatively healthy one.

Unfortunately, part of the difficulty in counseling people with hepatitis C is that it progresses with different symptoms and at different rates for different individuals. More research needs to be done to better understand the natural course of hepatitis C infection in a broad range of infected people. We are now developing ways that may allow us to counsel individuals better about their risks for progression of the infection and at what rate the infection will progress.

The primary information used for this risk assessment is the liver biopsy, interpreted by a pathologist. Naturally, the better the pathologist, the more accurate the prediction is likely to be. These liver biopsies are best interpreted by pathologists who routinely analyze liver biopsies from individuals infected with hepatitis C. The liver biopsy may show minimal, moderate, or robust inflammation. This may correspond with the degree of aggressiveness of the infection at the moment of the biopsy. The most important information obtained via liver biopsy is the severity of liver disease at the time of liver biopsy. There can be scarring or fibrosis in the liver, and this is one of the more important markers for prognosis. Naturally, if the liver is already markedly scarred over, compatible with cirrhosis, this is not a good sign. Fibrosis, however, may be leading up to cirrhosis but fall just short of it; it may be moderate, or minimal. The degree of fibrosis is a direct interpretation of the degree of permanent damage to the liver at the time of liver biopsy. So, both the degree of active inflammation and the degree of fibrosis need to be assessed as the liver biopsy is interpreted.

The liver biopsy is generally performed as an outpatient procedure. The person anticipating liver biopsy has his platelet count and serum clotting factors checked prior to the procedure, because the most frequent complication of liver biopsy is bleeding. Once an adequate platelet count and adequate clotting time have been documented, a liver biopsy is performed after discussing risks, benefits, and alternatives with the person preparing for the biopsy. The individual lies down on his back and places his right arm behind his head. The liver is identified by percussion which involves tapping on the individual's side to confirm the liver's location. The skin and space between the ribs are numbed with lidocaine. This anesthetic can cause a stinging sensation much like an insect bite or bee sting. Sometimes, when the needle is inserted, the person being biopsied can feel a pressure in the right arm. This is known as referred pain, or pain that derives from a site other than that in which it is perceived. Another example of this is phantom limb pain, in which someone who has undergone an amputation perceives pain in the leg that is no longer present.

The liver biopsy is done at full expiration (i.e., emptiest state of the lungs), and cooperation between the physician performing the liver biopsy and the patient is critical at this juncture. The person being biopsied is instructed to take a deep breath in and exhale completely, holding his diaphragm still in a fully exhaled position. The liver biopsy needle is inserted just above a rib, and then further inserted in the liver and quickly withdrawn to obtain a small sample of liver. This liver sample is generally 2–5 cm in length. Occasionally it is necessary to make more than one pass with the needle if an adequate biopsy sample is not obtained on the first pass. The person then must lie on his side for approximately 4–6 hours to allow adequate time for bleeding to stop. (This pressure over the biopsy site is like holding pressure on a cut to stop bleeding.) After being observed in the recovery area, he is allowed to go home if no problems are detected. If he feels lightheaded or dizzy after going home, it is critical that he be taken to the nearest emergency room for evaluation to be sure that he is not experiencing bleeding inside his abdomen after the liver biopsy.

Other, less frequent complications from liver biopsy include nicking the lung with the liver biopsy needle, infection or puncture of an intestine or part of the biliary tree or gallbladder. Most of these complications are routinely handled with either medical or surgical intervention. If the individual is quite ill, naturally these complications pose a greater risk and can even very rarely be life threatening. Nevertheless, in over 98% of people, a liver biopsy is performed without any adverse consequence, and the information obtained is integral to the individual's health care and prognosis.

Most people undergoing a liver biopsy experience a great deal of anxiety during the procedure. Because of the need for cooperation, sedation is generally not given, and the individual must control his anxiety by rational understanding and force of will. Working together as a team is essential to minimize risks. People may experience discomfort at the site of needle insertion, or referred pain in the form of a pressure in the right arm at the time of needle insertion. Having to lie still on one's side for 4–6 hours can also cause a great deal of discomfort for those with arthritis or back problems. Nevertheless, it is important to recognize that in an otherwise healthy person, liver biopsy is generally a safe and routine part of medical care of the individual with liver disease. The risks associated with the procedure are significant, but it is considered safe compared to the other option, which is doing without the valuable information that only a biopsy can yield.

HEPATOCELLULAR CARCINOMA

As Dr. Bates tried to explain hepatocellular carcinoma to Rudy, he interrupted. "I am an engineer. I need to see a picture to understand what the heck is going on. Show me a picture of what you mean about this liver cancer." Dr. Bates flipped over a clean sheet of paper. On it, he drew a sketch of a normal liver. Next, he drew an arrow signifying the introduction of the hepatitis C virus into the liver. Next, he drew a picture of a second, shrunk-down, nodular, scarred liver, representing cirrhosis. He drew a line from the first liver to the cirrhotic one with the overlying note, "years to decades." Finally, he drew a third liver, also shrunken, scarred, and nodular, but this time with a big "mass," or tumor, in it. He drew another arrow connecting the cirrhotic liver with the cirrhotic liver containing the tumor. Over this line, he wrote "3% incidence of tumor per year."

Dr. Bates then discussed the important issues of preventing hepatocellular carcinoma by treating people with chronic hepatitis C as well as screening for hepatocellular carcinoma in the context of cirrhosis and chronic hepatitis C. The exact mechanism by which hepatitis C virus causes hepatocellular carcinoma, or liver cancer, is not well defined. We know that once a person becomes cirrhotic there is approximately a 1–3% chance per year of developing hepatocellular carcinoma, compared to a negligible risk in the noncirrhotic population. The likelihood of developing hepatocellular carcinoma therefore increases with the length of time one has been infected with hepatitis C with cirrhosis. Therefore, eliminating hepatitis C virus from the body or preventing the development of

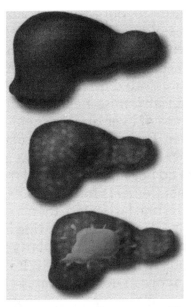

Figure 3. Hepatocellular carcinoma, liver cancer. The top panel shows the normal appearance of the liver. As the liver becomes cirrhotic, copious fibrosis or scar tissue is deposited throughout the organ, and it usually becomes shrunken in size and nodular as opposed to smooth in contour (middle panel). When it grows, liver cancer associated with hepatitis C usually occurs after cirrhosis has set in. The bottom panel depicts a scarred-over, shrunken, nodular liver that has developed a liver tumor in its midst. The liver, which became cirrhotic from hepatitis C infection, has an increased risk of developing liver cancer. This occurs at a rate of 1–3% per year. If someone lives with a cirrhotic liver for 10 years, the risk of developing liver cancer might be 10–30%.

cirrhosis secondary to hepatitis C virus infection is of the utmost importance in cancer prevention. Screening for hepatocellular carcinoma may be done through imaging studies of the liver, including liver ultrasound, as well as drawing α-fetoprotein levels (pronounced ALFA-FEE-TA-PROTEIN). α-Fetoprotein is a protein produced during the development of the human fetus, but before birth it stops being produced in detectable quantities. As cells in the liver turn into cancers, approximately 80% of hepatocellular cancers will register once again.

This is a useful marker to follow, but is not reliable all the time. There are instances of people with quite large hepatocellular carcinomas but with normal α-fetoprotein levels. Therefore approximately 20% of patients with hepatocellular carcinoma will not display an elevated α-fetoprotein level.

Ultrasound can also miss hepatocellular carcinoma formation. The presence of liver tumors should be investigated if an individual's liver disease abruptly worsens.

Fortunately, hepatocellular carcinomas grow rather slowly. Unfortunately, we do not have very good treatments for most of them. Current requirements for liver transplant listing would include that there be one lesion less than 5 cm or three lesions less than 3 cm in size. Nevertheless getting a liver donation for transplantation is problematic, particularly in states where the wait for a liver tends to be very lengthy. It is of critical importance to realize that organ donation rates vary from one state to another, and even from one organ procurement region to another within a given state. Inner-city neighborhoods, where trust of physicians and access to healthcare are often low, tend to have lower donation rates than communities with more aggressive health care. Unfortunately, it seems that the most common reason for missed opportunities to donate an organ is that the bereaved relatives or patient prior to death were never asked to help someone else. This is changing with time, but not fast enough for the thousands of patients who will die on organ waiting lists this year.

With regard to chemotherapy for hepatocellular carcinoma, the currently available drug regimens would have to be viewed as experimental. Anyone embarking upon treatment of hepatocellular carcinoma should consider treatment under an approved trial drug protocol. Radiation therapy is not often employed either, although both may be used as adjuncts to protocols in treating large tumors. The most common method of controlling hepatocellular carcinoma growth involves injecting the tumor with 100% alcohol, which kills at least a portion of the tumor tissue, allowing the body to replace the tumor with scar tissue. This can slow progression of the disease. Another method involves inserting a probe into the liver to kill the tumor with high-frequency radio waves, which generate heat and burn the tumor itself. This can be quite effective in slowing the progression of these tumors, although one should not be optimistic that either of these measures would cure the disease.

The only present method to cure hepatocellular cancer is to remove it surgically, either by cutting out a slice of liver containing the tumor or by removing the entire tumor at the time of liver transplantation. Surgical resection, cutting out a piece of liver, is an option if the tumor is accessible and the remaining liver could provide sufficient functional reserve. Assuming that postsurgical liver function would remain adequate, the liver section containing the tumor sometimes is approachable for partial liver resection to remove the tumor. Naturally, this procedure is not without risk, as a person with underlying cirrhosis is at increased risk for worse liver function due to the stress of removing part of the liver. Normally, the healthy part of the liver may compensate for the removed section. If the remaining liver is diseased, it is harder for this piece of liver to grow and carry out the job of the liver part removed at surgery. Resection may also fail to remove all of the tumor, allowing the targeted cells to proliferate and undo the effect of the surgery. Occasionally very superficial or peripheral lesions can be easily resected with lobectomy (removal of one of the liver's lobes) or a partial wedge resection (removal of only part of a lobe). Unfortunately, tumors, even when small, can often be buried so deep in the liver organ as to make resection an impossibility.

Liver disease specialists have not reached a consensus about the screening for hepatocellular carcinoma. Some screen by means of abdominal ultrasounds every 12 months and measurement of serum α-fetoprotein levels every 6 months, but this has not been shown in a randomized trial to improve longevity or outcome. The costs and inconvenience to the individual of this kind of regimen can be quite substantial, and in the absence of strong, compelling evidence of benefit, many physicians elect to screen for hepatocellular carcinoma only when an individual's liver disease symptoms progress to the stage of decompensation.

The use of screening tests for hepatocellular carcinoma might increase if there were better treatments for this disease. The point of finding tumors is to treat them; therefore, there is less reason to screen for less treatable tumors. Screening might also be more appealing if the methods were better: currently available tests miss too many tumors. Finally, the best approach to hepatocellular carcinoma at present is to be proactive and prevent its formation. This involves removing inciting agents, such as hepatitis C infection, which are known to predispose patients to the development of liver cancer (hepatocellular carcinoma). Other agents which can lead to the development of hepatocellular carcinoma include anything that causes cirrhosis, such as excess alcohol consumption.

One other known culprit in causing hepatocellular carcinomas is hepatitis B infection. One distinction between hepatitis B and hepatitis C is that hepatitis B can cause hepatocellular carcinoma either before cirrhosis has set in or after, and hepatitis C generally does not cause hepatocellular carcinoma until cirrhosis has occurred. Another noteworthy aspect of hepatitis C infection involves the presence of viral proteins in the liver for prolonged periods of time. It has been hypothesized that some of these proteins act as oncogenes, genes that stimulate cells to grow and divide more often than they otherwise would. It is the presence of such oncogenes that might lead to liver tumor formation. This may be a mechanism for the formation of liver tumors, although this has not been definitely proven, either through experimental laboratory studies or through clinical studies of patients who develop this disease.

Chronic hepatitis C infection may run its course to cirrhosis over years or decades. Some individuals infected with hepatitis C may never develop cirrhosis, as other diseases may affect them before the hepatitis C infection has had enough time to fully scar the liver. Even those without cirrhosis may develop symptoms of fatigue, abdominal pain, and loss of energy. Once the liver is scarred with cirrhosis, over time there is a decreased life expectancy caused by liver disease in comparison to people without cirrhosis. The virus can be cured in some cases, and it is therefore important to identify those individuals who are infected and eligible for current treatments. It is also important to identify infected individuals to help stem the spread of the virus through exposure to contaminated blood. There are several serum tests to detect the virus, and liver biopsy may be useful in confirming the diagnosis as well as assessing a particular individual's risk from liver disease.

4

Hepatitis C and End-Stage Liver Disease

Hepatitis C can lead to cirrhosis, or scarring over, of the liver and, ultimately, end-stage liver disease in the form of decompensated cirrhosis. The symptoms of decompensated cirrhosis include encephalopathy (confusion), ascites (fluid retention in the belly), swelling of the ankles, and gastrointestinal bleeding. Encephalopathy results from the buildup of toxic compounds normally cleared by the liver. Some of these toxins can impair brain function (hence the word "intoxication"). The symptoms of encephalopathy can vary from mild personality changes or difficulty to come up with the right word to express oneself all the way to frank coma. In between these extremes, people may have trouble remembering names, places, dates, or phone numbers. Short-term memory may be impaired. The ability to concentrate or do complex calculations may also decrease. Sleep disturbances, such as difficulty sleeping at night and taking brief, unfulfilling naps during the day, may also be signs of encephalopathy. Finally, worsening encephalopathy may manifest itself as severe exhaustion and lassitude, stuporous confusion, and ultimately hepatic coma, loss of consciousness. Fortunately, not all patients with end-stage liver disease wind up developing encephalopathy.

What determines who gets encephalopathy and who does not? The precise cause of encephalopathy is unknown but clearly correlates with worsening liver function. Worsening renal failure and constipation have been noted to worsen hepatic encephalopathy. External stresses may also worsen encephalopathy, such as infections, irregularities of serum salts or electrolytes, sleeping pills or pain medicines, excessive protein intake, and the protein load caused by gastrointestinal bleeding. If an individual bleeds into his stomach, the blood is broken down as it passes through the intestines. Partially digested proteins in the blood are reabsorbed into the circulation, placing an increased load on the liver. In patients prone to encephalopathy, a large gastrointestinal bleed may make the symptoms much worse. If someone suddenly develops markedly worse encephalopathy, it is important to look for a precipitating cause, such as infection, which may be treated.

How is hepatic encephalopathy treated? Lactulose, a non-absorbable sugar, helps loosen stools and may improve mentation. The antibiotics neomycin and metronidazole have also been used to treat encephalopathy with some success. Finally, depending on the individual beliefs of your physician, protein restriction in the diet may well be attempted.

Scarring of the liver can result in fluid accumulation as the scarring leads to pressure being exerted on the blood that normally passes through the liver, as well as decreased production of serum proteins. Serum proteins, you will recall, provide a broad range of functions including helping to hold fluid inside of the blood vessels in the body and prevent it from weeping out of blood vessels into the abdomen or subcutaneous tissues of the lower extremities. The combination of increased pressure pushing fluid out of blood vessels and decreased proteins holding fluid inside blood vessels leads to fluid leaking out of the blood system and accumulating inside the abdomen (ascites). Once present in the abdomen, this fluid is susceptible to infection and can require drainage at times as well as the use of diuretics (medicines that increase volume of urination). The importance of following a salt-restricted diet in the setting of fluid accumulation in the abdomen cannot be overstated.

End-stage liver disease affects the kidneys. The changes in the blood flow that result from liver failure increase salt retention by the kidneys. Fluid is retained along with salt, leading to a total body fluid overload. As a result, people infected with hepatitis C who have already developed end-stage liver disease frequently require diuretics or medicines which make them urinate and lose salt through the kidneys.

Hepatitis C infection is a leading cause of end-stage liver disease in this country and thus the primary necessitator of liver transplantation. End-stage liver disease occurs after the liver is scarred over or cirrhotic. End-stage liver disease (ESLD) can be defined as the time in a patient's liver disease when decompensated or unstable cirrhosis has set in. At this time liver transplantation may be under consideration. Symptoms include muscle wasting, fatigue, ascites, encephalopathy, or variceal bleeding. The vast majority of people with cirrhosis have compensated cirrhosis. "Compensated" means that the liver is scarred over but continues to function well, and the hepatitis C-infected individual experiences little if any adverse consequences of his cirrhosis. This is also known as a silent, or quiescent, cirrhosis. On the other hand, cirrhosis has more prominent symptoms in end-stage liver disease. These can include fatigue, disruption of the sleep–wake cycles, confusion or encephalopathy from the buildup of toxic compounds in the blood, ascites and accumulation of fluid in the ankles, muscle wasting, a failure to thrive or, more strikingly, bleeding from dilated blood vessels in the esophagus or stomach known as varices. The liver usually functions to remove toxic compounds from the body. When these compounds are allowed to build up in the body, they can, as has been noted, cause confusion. This confusion can be mild, in the form of difficulty remembering names, places, or facts. People suffering from more severe encephalopathy, however, may become so confused that they fail to recognize loved ones, lose their way back to their home, or have difficulty finding the bathroom. In its severest manifestations encephalopathy can progress to coma.

Ascites has several potential causes and effects. Decreases in the proteins made by the liver cavity may contribute to ascites by allowing fluid to seep out of the blood vessels and into the abdomen. Other potential causes include scarring over of the liver, leading to an increase in portal pressure. The portal vein carries blood from the gut to the liver. When the liver is scarred over, the pressure inside this vein increases, and this can force fluid into the abdomen. This ascitic fluid basically serves as a culture medium or food for bacteria, providing a source of energy and a warm, hospitable environment for the bacteria to grow. The source of bacterial seeding of the ascites can either be dental problems (such as poor dental hygiene) or urinary seeding of the ascites from an infected bladder. Either of these possibilities should be considered when an individual develops spontaneous bacterial peritonitis (SBP). Many hepatologists place people with ascites on antibiotics to try to prevent infections of the urinary tract that may spread to the fluid in the abdomen. These are often rotated to prevent the development of antibiotic-resistant strains, because the occurrence of spontaneous bacterial peritonitis is a poor prognostic indicator for the outcome of liver disease. This means that once a patient has an episode of SBP, his likelihood of dying in the next year may be as high as 50%.

Gastrointestinal bleeding is a common complication of liver disease. What is gastrointestinal bleeding? Gastrointestinal bleeding is frightening because it occurs inside of us, in the food pipe or esophagus, stomach, small or large bowel. This internal bleeding may be a relatively minor annoyance, like a dripping faucet, or a cataclysmic proclamation of impending disaster, like a burst water main. It is important to recognize gastrointestinal bleeding and deal with it appropriately.

Since the bleeding is going on inside the body, the first notice of a problem may be bright red blood or partially digested blood leaking or gushing from one of the body orifices, the mouth or anus. Gastrointestinal bleeding is not necessarily painful, as we do not always sense pain inside our body in the same way we would sense a cut on our arm, for example. The source of gastrointestinal bleeding is usually identified by a detailed analysis of exactly what symptoms are accompanying the bleeding and endoscopic inspection of the upper or lower gastrointestinal tract. The upper tract consists of the stomach, food pipe or esophagus, and beginning of the small bowel or duodenum. Symptoms that would lead one to suspect brisk upper gastrointestinal bleeding include throwing up bright red blood. This kind of bleeding is obvious; if it happens, the nearest emergency room is where you belong as soon as possible. When the blood sits in the stomach for a while, clots can form. Sometimes people toss up dark blood clots. If the blood sits there long enough, it may become partially digested. When this happens, the blood takes on the appearance of coffee grounds, the stuff left in the filter after brewing a fresh pot of coffee. Finally, perhaps the most subtle evidence of upper gastrointestinal bleeding involves the passing of dark black stool, the color of a black asphalt road.

There are several potential sources of upper gastrointestinal bleeding, including ulcers (disruptions in the lining of the esophagus, stomach or small bowel), diffuse mucosal bleeding (blood weeping diffusely across the lining of the stomach), and variceal bleeding (blood leaking out of large dilated blood vessels which can line the esophagus and stomach in the setting of liver disease). Ulcers affect about 1:10 Americans throughout their lifetime. Ulcers are the most common cause of bleeding in patients without liver disease, and may cause one-third of upper gastrointestinal bleeding even in patients with advanced liver disease. Ulcers are often accompanied by gnawing, intermittent upper abdominal pain, particularly between meals and late at night. The two most common causes of ulcers are aspirinlike drugs called nonsteroidal anti-inflammatory drugs (NSAIDs) and a bacterium known as *H. pylori*. It is best if patients with serious liver disease avoid NSAIDs including aspirin, ibuprofen, ketoprofen, and naproxen. Other agents that may exacerbate ulcers include alcohol, steroids, and anticoagulants such as coumadin or heparin. Ulcers can lead to further complications if left unattended. In addition to bleeding and pain, ulcers can eat right through the stomach or small-bowel wall, leading to a perforation of the digestive tract if left untreated. Scarring caused by an endless cycle of injury and healing may lead to obstruction of the gastrointestinal tract, which may manifest by vomiting and early fullness after eating.

When an ulcer is identified as the source of bleeding, it is important to consider NSAID use as a possible cause. Alternative pain medications are available that do·not attack the gastrointestinal tract quite as aggressively. Biopsies, blood or breath tests may be performed to assess for the presence of *H. pylori*, the bacterium that has been identified to cause the majority of ulcers. When *H. pylori* sets up its home in the stomach of many individuals, recurrent ulceration ensues. Fortunately, antibiotics can be used to get rid of this important pathogen and break the cycle of recurrent ulcer formation.

In patients with advanced liver disease and significant upper intestinal bleeding, the source of bleeding is an ulcer one-third of the time, a bleeding varix another third of the time, and diffuse mucosal (stomach lining) bleeding the final third of the time. In order to differentiate among different sources of bleeding, upper endoscopy is often performed. This involves using a fiberoptic instrument, which looks like a long, flexible black hose about the diameter of an adult index finger, to look inside of the upper gastrointestinal tract. The endoscope has a tiny fiberoptic light and microscopic camera built into its end which permit visualization of the upper gastrointestinal tract. When there is significant upper gastrointestinal bleeding this test is used to inspect the tract and look for a source of the bleeding so that appropriate therapy may be taken.

Signs of bleeding from the lower gastrointestinal tract, the small and large bowel, and rectum include passing bright red- or partially coagulated maroon-colored blood with or mixed into the stool. Occasionally, pure blood may gush from the anus. Sources of lower gastrointestinal bleeding also include ulcers (breaks in the lining of the lower tract), varices (engorged veins) or hemorrhoids, fissures, and polyps or growths in the colon. The source of lower gastrointestinal bleeding may also be evaluated by endoscopy—either colonoscopy or flexible sigmoidoscopy. Bleeding may be a sign of cancer, diverticuli or pouches in the bowel, as well as abnormal interminglings of the arterial and venous blood supply to the gastrointestinal tract known as arteriovenous malformations, or AVMs.

The sources of gastrointestinal bleeding that are almost unique to people with liver disease are varices and portal gastropathy. What are varices and how do they form? When pressure in the portal vein increases, the blood also starts to find circuits through the body other than through the liver. These pathways generally involve dilatation ·of small veins which already exist. These dilated veins are called varices and can develop in the esophagus, stomach, and bowels. They generally develop in the bottom part of the esophagus, where it meets the stomach, or in the top part of the stomach, where it meets the esophagus. Varices may also be present farther down, in the small bowel and in the colon. The most common sources of variceal bleeding are esophageal and gastric varices. The varices have thin walls and carry large volumes of blood at higher-than-normal pressure. When these varices break, profuse bleeding can occur. Blood can then come pouring into the stomach; as much as a gallon or two of blood may accumulate in the stomach or be expired by projectile vomiting. Understandably, this can be quite frightening to individuals infected with hepatitis C, their family members, and healthcare workers. It is not infrequent for people with variceal bleeding to pass out. Other times, these people with bleeding varices may pass a great deal of blood clots or black, partially digested blood (known as melena) into the toilet. If any of these signs are observed in a person with liver disease, it is imperative that he or she obtain medical attention immediately. For the patient suffering from variceal bleeding, it is reassuring to know that varices can be treated by several different approaches.

One of the methods used to treat varices involves banding. Banding is done with an endoscope, a fiberoptic instrument about the diameter of an adult's index finger which has a camera with light source on the end. The throat is numbed and the individual receives conscious sedation and then swallows the endoscope. This procedure, which visualizes the inside of the esophagus, stomach, and early part of the small intestine, enables the doctor to diagnose the source of the bleeding. If the bleeding is from an ulcer, stomach cells (gastropathy), or gastric varices, treatments may be quite different from treatments for bleeding from esophageal varices. If the bleeding is from esophageal varices, it is possible to perform banding to stop the bleeding. Banding involves sucking up a portion of the esophageal vessels and mucosa against the endoscope and then placing a specially designed, medical rubber band around them through the endoscope. This rubber band clots off the bleeding and stops it. The tissue caught in the rubber band dies and scars over, forming a strong wall which can prevent or diminish the possibility of further variceal bleeding. Generally it is necessary to perform band ligation more than once to obliterate esophageal varices, often in several different visits a few weeks apart.

Another treatment for varices involves sclerotherapy, the injection of fluid around or into the varix to cause pressure on the varix and necrosis of the tissue leading to scar formation. Sclerotherapy is performed using an endoscope, a device that allows us to look inside the food pipe and see the varices. Through a small channel in the endoscope, a catheter with a needle at the end is inserted. The needle is then pushed through the varix, and the sclerosant is injected. Sclerosants are the injected fluids which may include salt water or a variety of chemicals which induce scar formation.

Medical treatment can also be effective in managing varices. For acute bleeding, medicines such as vasopressin, somatostatin, and nitrates may be used to cause vasospasm (constriction of the blood vessels) and decrease the amount of blood flowing through the portal system, thereby diminishing bleeding from varices. More chronically, agents that reduce blood flow to the gut and through the liver may be used, such as the beta blocker propranolol.

Shunt surgery may be employed to relieve the pressure in swollen blood vessels (varices) in the esophagus, stomach, and other parts of the digestive tract. As has been discussed, these vessels are swollen because they are connected to the blood vessels that course through the liver. As the liver scars over, the pressure in these vessels increases, predisposing them to bleeding. By relieving the pressure in these swollen vessels, it is possible to stop bleeding from varices and prevent future bouts of variceal bleeding. Shunts may be either operatively placed by a surgeon or angiographically placed by an invasive radiologist to move blood flow away from or through the liver and relieve the pressure on the engorged varices. Over 50 years ago, surgical shunts were the first type of shunts used. These portal systemic shunts involve an abdominal operation to connect the portal vein, which carries blood flow into the liver, with the large vein, which carries blood back to the heart. This connection relieves pressure on the varices, but carries with it concomitant operative risks such as infection, intraoperative bleeding, and damage to other vital organs. Because people with advanced liver disease can be quite sick and fragile, this procedure is only appropriate for a small fraction of patients with variceal bleeding. When the procedure is performed on an emergency basis, when a patient is bleeding uncontrollably, the survival rate may be as low as 50%.

If successfully completed, the portal–systemic shunt prevents recurrent variceal bleeding yet it is seldom used today.

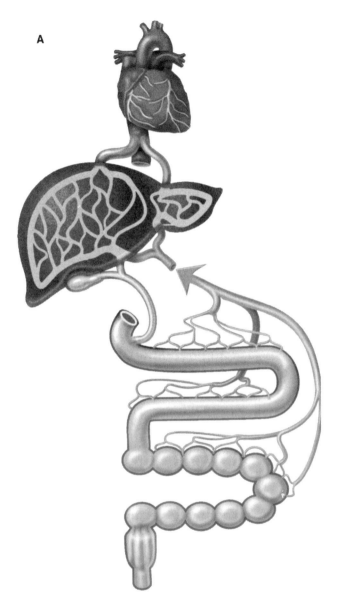

Figure 4.   See caption on page 56.

B

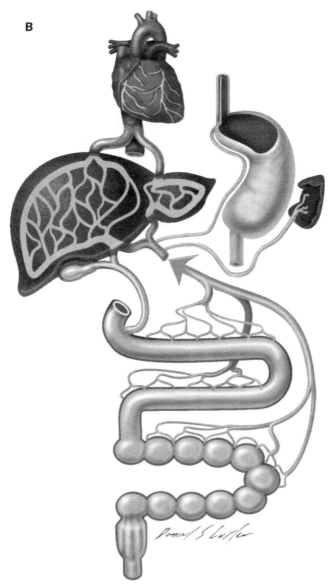

Figure 4.   See caption on page 56.

C

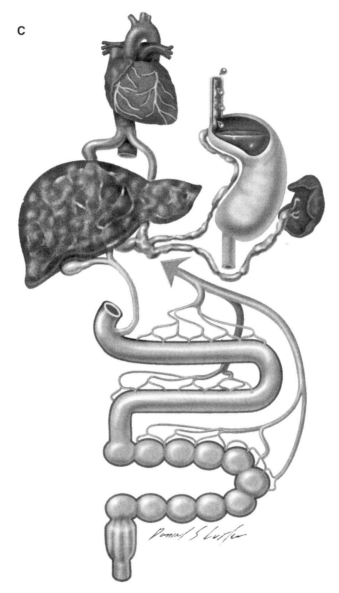

Figure 4.   See caption on page 56.

D

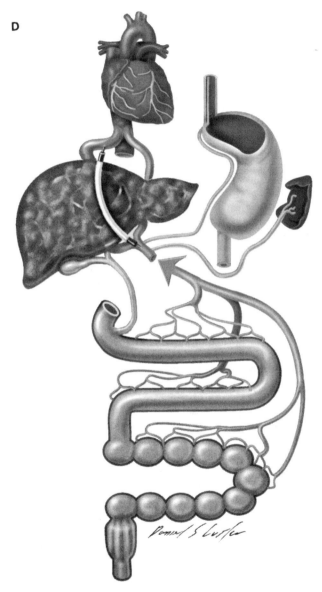

Figure 4.   See caption on page 56.

Shunt surgery may make liver transplant surgery more difficult or in some cases impossible, as it may scar up areas the
surgeons need to access to perform the liver transplant. This
type of portal–systemic shunt surgery also carries with it a
markedly increased risk of developing or worsening hepatic
encephalopathy (confusion from liver dysfunction). As blood
flow is diverted away from the liver, the liver no longer functions as well to remove toxins from the body.

Figure 4.   Normal anatomy, esophageal varices and insertion of a TIPS
shunt. The liver has a lot of blood flowing through it normally chiefly from
the bowel (bottom), up through the liver (middle), and into the heart (top,
panel A). Normally, a small amount of the blood which comes from the
bowel is diverted to flow into the spleen, stomach, and esophagus or food
pipe as shown by the addition of these organs in the next panel to the right of
the liver in the middle of the illustration (panel B). As the liver becomes
sicker and more scarred over, the blood flowing from the bowel cannot make
it through the liver easily (panel C). The blood finds other places to flow. As
pressure builds up in the blood vessels leading into the liver, the blood
vessels expand and blood courses through dilated or engorged blood vessels
(varices) inside the esophagus and stomach. The spleen also enlarges as it
handles more blood, sometimes leading to pain in the abdomen. The thin-
walled vessels or blood pipes can pop if the pressure gets too great, leading
to copious bright red bleeding into the food pipe (esophagus) or stomach
(panel C). The individual who suffers variceal bleeding may then throw up
bright red blood, partially digested blood with the appearance of coffee
grounds, or may pass black, tarlike stools. The bleeding is shown in panel C
as large drops of blood spilling out of the food pipe into the stomach and up
and out of the top of the esophagus. This kind of bleeding, variceal bleeding,
is frightening. One treatment for bleeding from engorged vessels in the
stomach or food pipe is to insert a TIPS shunt through the liver (panel D).
Since the bleeding comes from too much blood flowing around the liver and
dilating blood vessels in the esophagus and stomach, one method of treating
this bleeding is to use a shunt or pipe to carry blood through the liver. This
keeps blood from flowing into the engorged blood vessels in the food pipe
and stomach, decompressing them or reducing their size. These TIPS shunts
are usually used either if it is not possible to control the bleeding by other
means or if the bleeding happens over again. The shunt is like a pipe that
carries blood up from the bowel through the scarred liver toward the heart.
Note that after the shunt is in place, the dilated vessels in the esophagus and
stomach shrink down, and the bleeding stops (panel D).

Alternative surgical and nonsurgical approaches to treating varices are favored. To address the problem of worsening encephalopathy or confusion, exhaustive efforts were expended to develop a shunt that maintained more of the blood flow to the liver while diverting blood flow away from bleeding engorged varices in the esophagus or stomach. This type of shunt has a long name which belies its nature: distal splenorenal shunt. In this procedure, one of the veins running to the spleen is hooked up to a vein running to the kidney, having the same effect as with earlier shunts to relieve pressure in engorged varices. Now, there is less encephalopathy or confusion after distal shunt surgery, while overall surgical risks persist. Yet studies of long-term survival showed that medical treatment of varices with drugs and sclerotherapy compared well with those receiving shunt therapy, so surgical therapy is reserved for highly select individuals who may have a favorable surgical benefit. Patients in whom surgical procedures are still used are those with problems from variceal bleeding who still maintain pretty good liver function and a robust overall medical condition predisposing them to a more favorable long-term survival. The advent of nonsurgically placed shunts has revolutionized the treatment of recurrent variceal bleeding.

Less invasive methods for performing shunts were sought owing to the difficult problems many patients experienced with shunt surgery. Radiologists developed what is known as a TIPS procedure—transjugular intrahepatic portosystemic shunt. The most striking advantages of this shunt procedure are its relative simplicity and the lack of stress for the bleeding individual. The invasive radiologist, a physician who specializes in performing tests and inserting stents with catheters under x-ray guidance, gives the person with variceal bleeding a moderate systemic sedative and local anesthetic in the neck where the needle is first inserted. The individual receiving the sedative remains conscious throughout the procedure, avoiding the risks of general anesthesia which is less well tolerated by people with liver disease. The TIPS shunt involves inserting a catheter through the jugular vein in the neck—through the major vein, the vena cava, down through the hepatic vein and actually poking a path through the liver with a needle inserted through the catheter. Fortunately, the liver does not sense pain the same way as your skin, so the passage of the needle through the liver is not an overtly painful sensation. Once the path is open across the liver, an inflatable balloon is used to open a wire mesh stent across the scarred liver. The stent is like a pipe that extends across the liver; this lowers the increased pressure created by the scarring and relieves the pressure on the engorged varices in the esophagus and stomach. There is now a pathway through the stent for blood to flow through the liver obviating the need for blood to seek its way through varices.

The TIPS procedure is generally performed in a matter of several hours in an angiography suite and does not involve an incision or abdominal operation. Because of its more rapid and less invasive nature, it is becoming one of the primary procedures performed to prevent recurrent or unstoppable bleeding from liver disease. In addition, the TIPS procedure leaves the individual free of an operative incision and scars which may hinder subsequent liver transplantation. Another major advantage of TIPS in comparison with surgical shunts is that the TIPS procedure can in many cases improve the fluid accumulation or ascites in the abdomen. In some cases, TIPS is used in an effort to manage ascites when diuretics and dietary modification have failed.

While TIPS procedures have been used with increasing frequency, they are not problem-free and significant risks should not be taken lightly. In experienced centers, the survival rate from the procedure is 95–98%, which means some people succumb even during this less invasive procedure. About 25% of individuals with liver disease who receive a TIPS develop worsening encephalopathy or confusion. Individuals with moderate to severe encephalopathy or weak heart function, which may not tolerate the increased blood load on the heart, may not be good candidates for the TIPS procedure. Similarly, TIPS must be used very carefully in patients with compromised kidney function. Finally, scar tissue often grows through or around the TIPS stent or pipe, causing it to get stopped up so that blood no longer flows through it properly. This is like a drain pipe getting stopped up and having a sink overflow leaking water on the floor. Instead of a sink overflowing, when a TIPS shunt gets blocked up, varices get increased pressure, potentially leading to a variceal bleed—blood pouring into the esophagus or stomach. People who receive TIPS shunts may need to have them cleaned of these obstructions or have them revised by reopening them with a balloon on the end of a catheter. People with TIPS shunts in place should usually have them checked carefully every 6 months to a year.

The success of TIPS is highly dependent on the physician who performs it. In general, TIPS procedures should be performed by physicians who perform enough of them each year to develop and maintain their competence. Naturally, repetition of a procedure gives a physician valuable experience; that alone does not assure competence, however. These special radiology doctors should be found at major referral centers which care for a significant number of individuals with end-stage liver disease.

The techniques to control variceal hemorrhage are in a continuous state of evolution. Medicine has advanced a long way from 50 years ago when there was little to offer individuals with variceal hemorrhage. Sclerotherapy, banding and medicines all are valuable tools in attempts to control variceal hemorrhage. When they fail to control variceal bleeding, the TIPS procedures can be an extremely valuable option. For selected patients with well-preserved hepatic function who are thought likely able to tolerate a surgical procedure, the distal splenorenal shunt remains an option to consider. Controlled trials comparing outcomes of different methods to manage variceal bleeding will lend further insight into how best to apply these various techniques. Ultimately, patients with end-stage liver disease should seek liver transplant evaluation, as ascites, variceal bleeding, encephalopathy (confusion), and muscle wasting are all warning signs of impending liver failure. Too often, sick people and their physicians wait too long to consider liver transplantation. With the inordinately long and growing wait on liver transplant lists, this can be an unfortunate circumstance. For those who are interested in considering a liver transplant, it is much better to request a liver transplant evaluation and be proclaimed too healthy than to delay and discover transplant was considered too late. If you have end-stage liver disease with muscle wasting, ascites, variceal bleeding or confusion (encephalopathy), you need not worry about losing credibility by going to get more information about a liver transplant too early. Most transplant centers are happy to follow patients for several years if necessary before listing. No one minds telling someone they are too healthy to meet liver transplant listing criteria. It is tragic to deal with someone who comes seeking help too late when a lengthy transplant list precludes a successful outcome. Increased organ donations may obviously help this situation as well.

5

Hepatitis C and Liver Transplantation

Dr. Bates next saw Rudy in the liver transplantation evaluation clinic. Rudy needed a new liver and was determined to get one. First, Bates explained that being placed on the transplant list required a thorough evaluation, and then a long wait lay ahead. Though Rudy was scared, he could also feel life's energy slipping from him every day. He sensed that he did not have long left if he did not get a liver transplant soon. He hoped he could make it.

Rudy was worried about finding a suitable donor who would provide a good match for him. He had seen fliers in the supermarket in which anxious families looked for bone marrow donors to match their loved one. He wondered how difficult the matches were for liver donor and recipient. He was afraid to ask about these things because he found the whole process overwhelming. Dr. Bates volunteered that liver donor–recipient matches are much simpler than bone marrow or kidney donor–recipient matches. Rudy was relieved to hear even a thread of good news. It turns out that while other tissues may be matched using a variety of tissue compatibility markers, livers are matched chiefly for blood type A, B, O, or AB. Ironically, while blood type AB is the rarest in the population, people with this blood type also generally have the shortest wait to get a donor organ. Blood type O usually has the longest wait, followed by type A and type B.

Liver transplantation is degenerating into a surreal lottery in which a new organ and the promise of renewed life are the ultimate prize. This has resulted from a severe shortage of donor livers, necessitating a prolonged wait on the liver transplant waiting list. Not all people who need a liver can get one. It is best to approach the process of liver transplant listing forewarned and armed with knowledge. You should know what keeps people off the list and what gets them on.

First, there are medical conditions that can preclude transplantation. If you have untreatable metastatic cancer, you cannot get a lottery ticket (a place on the liver transplant waiting list). If you have heart failure, particularly right-sided heart failure, you will probably not be able to survive the transplant, and you are not likely to be offered a place on the transplant list. Similarly, if you have pulmonary hypertension (increased pressure in the blood vessels leading into the lungs), the operation is not likely to be a success, and a place on the transplant list is not likely. Prior abdominal operations may slow the surgeon down or, in rare cases, lead to excessive scarring which makes the operation impossible.

Next, there are potential social and psychological barriers. If you have been drinking alcohol in the last 6 months, you won't be offered a spot if there is any chance alcohol use contributed to your liver disease. Since even small amounts of alcohol may multiply the damage from hepatitis C, alcohol use is a concern for any infected individual. If you are of advanced age, it is best to be robust and well preserved. If you smoke marijuana, be aware that it can take months to clear it from the body of someone with liver failure. Use of any recreational drugs is felt to predict relapse to alcohol, so drug screens including cocaine, narcotics, and marijuana had better turn up negative. Be prepared to submit to random drug and alcohol screens while on the waiting list. If alcohol has caused a large part of your problem, be prepared to admit this to yourself and others. Be prepared to attend alcohol rehabilitation if this is deemed beneficial. Multiple suicide attempts may keep you off the list. If there is a history of suicide attempts, better if they were gestures in the distant past rather than serious attempts to take your life. Family and friend support is important. If you are flat on your ass sick after the transplant, will someone care enough to bring you to the hospital? If you cannot keep track of your immunosuppressive medications, will someone organize them for you and help you take them? Will you keep your follow-up appointments? If the immunosuppressive medications give you a headache or change your appearance, are you likely to take them? It is necessary to take the immunosuppressive medications to prevent liver transplant rejection, even if there are deleterious side effects.

Nevertheless, the toxicities of immunosuppressive medications are not to be taken lightly. First, cyclosporine can raise blood pressure, cause loss of potassium, and trigger depletion of kidney function. The blasted medicine which makes organ transplantation possible can actually cause renal failure! Blood levels of the drug may vary widely, so they must be checked often. Over time, prednisone can cause thinning of the bones, which then fracture easily. There also may be hair loss and unwanted body fat deposition. Imuran can be teratogenic (cause fetal deformities). Immunosuppression also makes people more susceptible to opportunistic infections. These are infections the body normally handles routinely but which can attack the body when immune defenses are lowered by medicines that allow the organ transplantation to persist.

Liver transplantation is especially important for people with chronic hepatitis C infection with end-stage liver disease. Liver transplantation is now an accepted, routine medical procedure which is funded by most legitimate health insurance policies and Medicaid. The practice has been driven by the development of effective surgical techniques for transplantation and immunosuppressives which prevent the recipient from rejecting the donor organ, not to mention the altruism of those who, at the time of tragedy, elect to donate the gift of life to someone who needs a new liver. At present, over 4000 liver transplants are performed annually in the United States. Yet, estimates are that this covers only a small fraction of the people who would benefit from liver transplants. Unfortunately, the process of liver transplantation is limited by the availability of donor organs. Liver donors must meet certain set requirements. These can include brain death prior to organ donation, the absence of cancer or other, transmissible diseases and a healthy liver.

Unfortunately, many people who would be willing to donate organs do not, for a variety of reasons, the most common being that they have not been asked. Many states are now requiring that at the time of driver's license renewal people be asked if they are willing to donate their organs at the time of death. This simple inquiry will increase the supply of livers available. Even given these strategies, however, it is estimated that the potential demand for liver transplantation far outstrips the potential supply. Only brain-dead people are potential organ donors. Those who die from infection or cancer are not suitable donors as they might transmit disease to the recipient—the liver must be healthy.

The shortage of healthy livers for transplantation leads to the rationing of livers for transplantation on both the local and national levels. Nationally, there is an organization called UNOS which sets certain rules and conditions for the allocation of organs to liver transplantation centers. Each liver transplantation center has a liver transplant evaluation committee. People who sit on this committee make every effort to place people on the liver transplant waiting list equitably and fairly. The livers are allocated after a careful medical workup to exclude cardiovascular disease, pulmonary disease, malignancies and other conditions that might pose a risk of death at the time of liver transplantation or shortly thereafter. This evaluation can involve tests of cardiovascular reserve, including a stress test or even cardiac catheterization if the stress test reveals abnormalities. These selection issues are taken very seriously. Liver transplantation is one of the most stressful and intensive of surgeries. The physiologic stress placed on the individual receiving a liver graft is greater than the stress on an individual undergoing routine coronary artery bypass grafting.

Why are there so few organ donors? Current rules for organ donation in the state of Michigan, for example, restrict organ donation to brain-dead people whose heart is still beating. The focus on using heart-beating donors is to increase the probability that the organ is well perfused and healthy at the time of removal. This includes kidney, heart, lung, liver, pancreas, and intestine donors. While the age of the donor is not an absolute restriction, organ donation is commonly restricted to donors within the newborn-to-75-year-old age range. Owing to the shortage of suitable donors, older individuals' organs are being used more routinely.

In Michigan, the evaluation process is the responsibility of the Transplantation Society of Michigan. Other states or regions within states have agencies that function similarly. There is a donation coordinator on call 24 hours a day. Michigan state law requires that organ and tissue donation be offered as an option to the families of all individuals who have died in the hospital. The donors must be brain dead and on mechanical respiratory support. It should be noted that tissue donation, such as eye lenses or heart valves, does not require brain death; all deaths are potentially acceptable. Cases of unexpected death which are referred to the medical examiner's office to exclude foul play are not automatically excluded from organ donation. If the individual's prior wishes and family wishes concur, the medical examiner may grant permission for organ donation.

At or near the time of death, patients' families will be approached with a request for organ or tissue donation. This can often be a difficult time to make a life-saving decision. Often at the time of acute grieving, it is difficult for a patient's family to discuss the different aspects of tissue donation, and the ball can get dropped. Naturally, it is ideal if a patient has discussed his wishes with his family prior to the time the decision needs to be made. One common concern is whether organ donation will interfere with a donor's appearance for a traditional funeral home viewing; the answer is no. Importantly, organ donation does not cost anything to the family or the deceased patient's estate. In the state of Michigan, all costs related to organ donor evaluation, maintenance and surgical recovery of organs are paid by the Transplant Society of Michigan, which in turn recovers costs from the organ recipient's insurance.

So what happens when someone agrees to donate his liver for transplantation? First, the donation coordinator at the transplant society is notified. The evaluation of donor suitability includes the definitive medical determination of brain death, patient's diagnosis, medical history, current lab values (to evaluate for systemic illness that could compromise organ health), blood type, and body weight. It is important to determine if the patient has cancer or systemic infection, as either may eliminate a donor from being a candidate. This information is then conveyed to the hospital transplant program listing the next suitable liver recipient on the transplant society's list.

The hospital transplant program may accept the organ, reject the organ, or ask for further information about the organ donor. Such information might include length of time on blood pressure supporting medicines, and concomitant infections. Occasionally a liver biopsy of the donor may be requested to assess the vitality of the donor liver. The organ donor is maintained on mechanical ventilation and medications to support blood pressure if necessary. In this way, the donor organ continues to be perfused with warm, oxygenated blood while the organ harvesting team is dispatched. Unless an organ-harvesting team is present in the donor's hospital, one is dispatched to the donor. This team leaves their home base as soon as possible, frequently in the middle of the night. The team travels quickly, by helicopter if weather and distance permit. Alternative modes of travel include fixed-wing aircraft, or if all air traffic is grounded or the donor is close by, ground ambulance transportation may be applied. It is not unusual for a harvesting team to drive through a blizzard or other inclement weather (that would leave most citizens homebound) to go harvest and retrieve a donor organ.

When they arrive at the hospital, where the brain-dead donor lies in wait, they can do a more thorough assessment of donor organ suitability. For example, they may open the patient and note excessive fatty infiltration of the liver. Fatty infiltration of the liver is particularly common in even moderately obese people. Just as excessive fat is distributed all over the body including the face, abdomen, buttocks, and extremities, some fat can be deposited within the liver itself. Usually this fatty deposition does not interfere with the liver's normal function while the organ donor is alive. Yet, experience has taught liver transplant specialists that organs that contain excessive fatty deposition do not engraft well. Evidently the fat interferes with the vitality of the organ during the time of harvest, transport, or reestablishment of blood flow through the organ. The transplant surgeon, who is a member of the organ procurement team, visually inspects the liver through an incision in the donor's abdomen. If excessive fat is visually appreciated or if there is a suggestion of scarring or fibrosis, the liver may be biopsied at this time to further assess organ viability.

The donor is also screened for infectious diseases such as HIV and viral hepatitis. HIV-infected individuals are generally excluded from organ donation. Some centers, however, are using livers from donors with a prior history of hepatitis B infection for transplantation into people whose livers have failed from chronic hepatitis B infection. Similarly, some centers use hepatitis C-infected donor livers for transplantation into hepatitis C-infected recipients. Since the recipient's viral hepatitis may infect the donated liver anyway, the benefits of expanding the pool of donor organs are felt to outweigh the detriments of using previously infected livers. Naturally, these decisions are made with the knowledge of the recipient and on a case-by-case basis, assessing both donor organ vitality and the urgency of a recipient's need for an organ.

Once the decision has been made to harvest a donor organ, the organ procurement team proceeds to attentively remove or harvest the donor liver. Great care is taken to ensure its preservation for incipient transplantation while respecting the organ donor's dignity and integrity. The liver is cautiously dissected, cutting the nerves and small-caliber vessels which connect it to the donor. The large-caliber vessels, the bile duct, portal vein, hepatic artery, and hepatic vein are carefully dissected so that they are removed with the donor organ. These vessels will be meticulously sewn to the recipient, allowing the donated organ to function under near-physiologic conditions in the organ transplant recipient. The liver is perfused with an organ preservation solution, most typically "Wisconsin" solution. This is a salt, sugar, and water solution named after the state where it was developed. The solution is run through the liver to flush out the blood cells. The liver is removed from the donor, placed in a cooler on ice, and transported to the liver transplant center. The liver can usually be used for a couple of days after harvest, but it is strongly preferred that the organ be transplanted as soon as possible. Liver graft survival rates are a function of time from harvest to grafting; the longer an organ has been harvested, the less likely it is to engraft properly and provide viable liver function in the liver transplant recipient.

Because of the shortage of suitable organ donors, not everyone who wants a liver transplant can get one. There is an extensive evaluation by a multidisciplinary transplant team, including a social worker who evaluates for a history of substance abuse, and the presence of suitable family or friend support. Postoperative abuse of alcohol has been associated with failure of transplanted livers. This can either be from direct alcohol toxicity to the liver or from inebriation leading to neglect of the transplanted organ. When people are drunk, they may neglect to take immunosuppressive medications or neglect to seek medical attention or keep follow-up appointments. The extensive social work evaluation includes a history of prior attempts at rehabilitation. Questions typically concern a prior history of drunken driving, difficulties in relationships caused by alcohol, and a history of abuse of other substances. Since abuse of substances such as marijuana is felt to be indicative of a potential for a relapse to alcoholism, most programs require abstinence from all recreational drugs at the time of transplant. In addition, the use of alcohol and other recreational drugs, including marijuana, is not allowed within 6 months of transplant listing. It is quite possible that many cases of what was deemed alcoholic cirrhosis in the past may have actually involved alcohol and hepatitis C. Now that we have reliable tests to check for hepatitis C, many people who have even just consumed several drinks a day may end up with end-stage liver disease when alcohol use and hepatitis C infection are coincident.

The transplant allocation of organs is done on the basis of a waiting list divided into several levels based on the severity and duration of liver disease. Most people with hepatitis C infection have chronic liver disease, although the degree of liver dysfunction may vary from one individual to another. Symptoms that should prompt people to seek liver transplant evaluation include confusion or encephalopathy, ascites that is difficult to control with diuretics, spontaneous bacterial peritonitis, or gastrointestinal bleeding from the rupture of varices in the stomach or esophagus.

Nevertheless, as advances are being made in liver transplantation techniques, there is an impending crisis due to the shortage of donor organs. The number of people on waiting lists is growing daily as is the number of people who die while on the waiting list. Reports of a governor in Pennsylvania and a baseball player in Texas receiving organs after only a short period of time on the waiting list raise conjecture about the fairness of the process of organ allocation. Most centers have taken great strides not only to make the process of organ allocation fair, but also to remove any public perception of unfairness. Nevertheless, when someone fails to get an organ and dies, it is easy to be suspicious of the whole process. Since organ donation is based on altruism, fair and equitable organ allocation is necessary for maintaining donor trust in the system. For these reasons, it is imperative that the pool of organ donors be increased to limit the number of people who are seeking liver transplantation who do not receive one, and that alternative sources of organs be made available. This may be possible either through using organs that were not felt to be previously useful, such as ones that were from ill donors or have other problems associated with them, or through harvesting organs from other species. Ultimately, these decisions are made on a case-by-case basis, although there is intensive ongoing research to try to develop an expanded pool of donor organs.

Rudy was careful to keep all of his follow-up appointments with Dr. Bates. He would come early and get his blood drawn. When he noticed a change in his condition, he would call the transplant nurse.

Death was no stranger to Rudy. He had once served on an 8-man team whose mission was to search and destroy in the jungle. He had "scored" 37 kills in Vietnam. In the past, they were the enemy; over time each of his victims turned into a person. On one particularly traumatic occasion in Vietnam, Rudy was standing behind his friend when the friend's head was blown clean off. The fragments of his friend's skull and brain showered across Rudy's chest, and Rudy understandably went berserk. They had to restrain him, sedate him, and take him out of that village by helicopter. Rudy still gets nauseated on the anniversary day of this event every year. As he got ready for his transplant, these images flashed through his head. He remembered the smell of the decaying carcasses as he stuffed them into body bags after a Marine camp was overrun in North Vietnam. That graveyard duty was the worst assignment he had pulled; he thanked God he had only had to do it for one week. He pulled himself together. After all he had been through, how bad could this liver transplant be? He was scared because the reality was that this time it was him. He was going to have his body opened, his liver was going to be removed, and someone else's liver was going to be sutured into place. He was determined to overcome his fear and succeed. He did not like the feeling that his fate was at least in part out of his control. He waited pensively for a donor.

As Rudy neared the top of the transplant list, he was provided with a long-range beeper so that he could be contacted when a liver became available. Three weeks later, Rudy's beeper went off while he was shopping for a new hat. The transplant coordinator was delighted yet somber; a young man had just donated a liver for Rudy. Rudy could feel his heart race. This was the big call, determinant of his future quality of life. He felt doubt for a moment; would he survive? Then he brushed it away, showered, and drove to the hospital. Time was racing. He checked in at admitting and donned his hospital gown. Again they drew his blood. Off he was whisked to the operating room. The anesthesiologist gave him something to chill his nerves, and that is the last he remembered until the recovery room.

Waking up, he felt all puffy. There was a large tube like a garden hose sticking out of his neck. "Jeez," he thought, "I feel like I gained 20 pounds during the operation." The next thing he noticed, however, was energy. He had not felt this good for several years. He could feel the rhythmic moving of his lungs as the ventilator moved air in and out of his lungs through an endotracheal tube passing from his mouth into his trachea. The next morning the nurses were turning Rudy over to clean him. He coughed the endotracheal tube out of his lungs and was breathing on his own. Dr. Bates came by to check in on Rudy. Dr. Bates told him the new liver was working well; he liked the color of Rudy's bile. No one had ever complimented Rudy's bile before, so he felt awkward, but tried to accept the compliment gracefully. He then remembered that it was not all *his* bile; for the first time he felt like a hybrid of two people. He could not articulate his thanks to the person who donated an organ so that he could carry on with his life.

Rudy went home 2 weeks after his surgery. He was feeling

well, walking and taking care of himself. Several days later, he turned bright yellow and lost his energy. He felt like a human banana. He had never been this yellow before. He called the transplant service, and they told him to come to the hospital immediately. He missed his hepatologist, Dr. Bates; there was a new team of doctors caring for him after his transplant. He did not understand why Dr. Bates could no longer care for him. They had grown rather close over the years. Fortunately, he liked his new doctors too. He did not know them well yet, and he was dealing with a lot of sudden changes. Now he was scared again. He felt more comfortable now that he was in the hospital again, but he did not like being there. Had this miracle of a new organ been plucked from him just as he was beginning to enjoy it?

Then a young doctor walked into his room. Rudy looked her over; he had a habit of forming a quick opinion of anyone who cared for him. This kid still had acne. She introduced herself as Dr. Hellen Shosha. She spoke comfortably and authoritatively, and this immediately put Rudy at ease. She explained that his new liver was not working as well as before he was discharged. They would need to run some tests, to be sure the bile duct was still open and that the blood vessels flowing into the liver were free from clots or narrowings. Next, should these prove unrevealing, they planned to do a liver biopsy to determine if he was suffering from "rejection." What an odd thought, that his body could be mounting an immune response to the new liver his mind welcomed so appreciatively.

After having several tests which were inconclusive, Dr. Shosha appeared at his bedside. She now explained that they were going to start treating him for rejection with a burst of intravenous steroids, and that she planned to do a liver biopsy. Shosha had done dozens of these biopsies before, but she always approached a liver transplant recipient with extra care. Within 3 minutes, she was telling Rudy to lie on his side for 6 hours. She wandered out of the room, telling Rudy tomorrow they would be able to look at his liver sample under a microscope to confirm the diagnosis of rejection. Rudy had been warned about rejection; he had just assumed it would not be a problem for him. The doctor told him that graft rejection occurred in 50–80% of liver transplants, resulting in failure of the graft 5–10% of the time. Besides acute rejection, which occurs shortly after liver transplant, there is also another, more chronic form of rejection which can occur many months to years after transplantation. Rudy thought he would like to avoid this type of rejection as well, but that was more of a future concern. Right now, he just wanted to go home.

Slowly, his skin color started to clear. His urine was no longer dark brown and his stool was no longer yellow. He could feel his energy returning. He remembered how he had been warned of all the side effects of the immunosuppressive medicines. These things had just saved his new liver. They were a necessary evil he was learning to appreciate. He was sent home in good spirits.

Several months later a neighbor of Rudy's, Mr. Green, came to see Dr. Bates. Mr. Green was a 72-year-old lawyer with bad coronary disease. He developed decompensated cirrhosis and was found to be infected with hepatitis C. He had suffered several heart attacks which had badly damaged his heart. In 1989, he underwent coronary artery bypass grafting (CABG) and received 6 units of blood during the operation. Mr. Green came to see Dr. Bates for liver transplant evaluation. When Dr. Bates told Mr. Green that his heart was too weak to get him through a liver transplant operation, Mr. Green cried. "You know, I think they gave me this virus when they gave me blood transfusions during the heart operation. Now there is no way to make up for it." Dr. Bates could not help but feel a pang of guilt; having ordered many blood transfusions before 1992, he had no doubt given several of his patients hepatitis C unintentionally. He reassured Mr. Green that they had no way of knowing then which units of the blood supply were contaminated with hepatitis C, and that every effort had been made to correct the problem once the virus was discovered. He also pointed out that medicine is an imperfect science, but mostly he tried to console Mr. Green. There was no good way for Dr.

Bates to say these things to Mr. Green, and Dr. Bates could only imagine how hard it must be to hear news like that.

In the face of the difficult news Mr. Green had received, he sulked out of the clinic. He wanted to sue someone for what had happened to him, but realized it was nobody's fault. He heard about a law suit in Canada, but found out that there the test to screen blood for hepatitis C had not been used even when it was available. Canadians had therefore received hepatitis C-tainted blood even when the test to exclude those units was available and could have prevented disease transmission. Briefly, Mr. Green wished he were Canadian. Eventually, Mr. Green consoled himself with the thought that liver transplantation might only be a temporary treatment for hepatitis C, as the virus can reinfect the new liver following transplantation. He was surprised to learn that over 70% of people with hepatitis C who undergo a liver transplant have hepatitis C-induced cirrhosis of the liver again 5 years after transplant.

Liver transplantation extends hope to people who have liver failure. When successfully applied, liver transplants may miraculously restore vigor and robust health. It is far from a certain science, and drug reactions, surgical complications, and opportunistic infections all serve to make the posttransplant course unpredictable. Long waiting lists and a shortage of donor organs make liver transplantation particularly problematic. Once signs of end-stage liver failure such as confusion, variceal bleeding, muscle wasting, and ascites set in, early requests for liver transplant evaluation are prudent.

6

Stopping the Spread of Hepatitis C

Blood Transfusions, Recreational Drug Use, Sex, Tattoos, Acupuncture, Manicures, Pedicures, and Body Piercing

The majority of hepatitis C virus infections are spread through blood contact. This may be in the form of blood transfusions, intravenous drug use, tattoos, acupuncture, manicures, pedicures, body piercing, or human bites. Rare forms of transmission may include sharing toothbrushes at the time of gingival bleeding, or bleeding at the time of sexual intercourse.

The contraction of hepatitis C as a result of transfusion is the result of one of the greatest disasters of modern medicine. Why has the medical community been so slow to come forth to the public with the details of hepatitis C infection? After all, physicians ordered the blood transfusions which in many cases resulted in the disease. Of course, the physicians meant well at the time and did not deliberately plot the spreading of hepatitis C. Since hepatitis C had yet to be identified, no one could screen for a disease which they didn't know existed. Yet, there has been a reluctance to admit any role the healthcare system played in the dissemination of hepatitis C. Similarly, there has been a lack of contrition on the part of the medical community for using contaminated blood. It is important that people trust their blood supply and are willing to receive blood transfusions if medically necessary. Similarly, it is crucial that patients trust their doctors. Nevertheless, it is only in 1999 that the Red Cross has started to notify all people who received blood transfusions prior to 1992 of their potential risk for hepatitis C infection.

Part of this delay has involved the complicated and varied course of hepatitis C infection which has only recently come to light. Part of this delay no doubt involves a component of denial on the part of the medical community to discuss publicly the dissemination of a potentially lethal infectious agent throughout the community as a result of a then-tainted blood supply. Are there other chronic viral infections that may be causing debilitating symptoms or shortening our lives? How can we screen for them if they are not yet identified? One way might be through surrogate disease markers.

Since we did not know what caused transfusion-related non-A, non-B hepatitis before the discovery of hepatitis C, one can ask if there was another way of figuring out which units of blood were at risk for transmitting the disease. One marker of hepatitis C infection in many, but far from all, individuals is elevated serum liver enzymes. Could the blood supply have been made safer if those units of blood coming from donors with elevated serum liver enzymes been discarded? At the time, probably at least one of every 100 units of blood was contaminated with hepatitis C. The practice of screening donor blood for elevated serum liver enzymes was adopted in 1986, resulting in the discard of 3% of all donated units of blood and cutting the subsequent risk of contracting transfusion-related hepatitis C by close to 50%. In retrospect, everyone wishes testing donated blood for serum liver enzymes had been practiced sooner; tens of thousands of hepatitis C infections could have been prevented.

How safe is the blood supply now?

Extremely. With modern blood tests for hepatitis C, the risk of getting hepatitis C from a blood transfusion in the United States is probably around 1 in 100,000. With regard to other chronic viral infections, we know of some viruses like hepatitis G, which is transmitted in blood. We have not been able to link this virus with any concrete disease so the blood supply is not routinely screened to eliminate it. *The best evidence available now*, and these things can change, is that hepatitis G is a benign agent which hangs around in people's blood and liver, like the barnacle on a ship. The unique aspect of hepatitis C infection was that posttransfusion hepatitis was a major concern before the blood supply was screened for hepatitis C, with up to 10% of those receiving transfusions developing inflammation of the liver. It should be noted that individuals receiving transfusions were often alerted to this risk prior to blood transfusion as well. The long-term effects of posttransfusion hepatitis were worse than appreciated at the time, because the symptom-free interval of infection with hepatitis C was so long that the adverse effects of the infection were probably underestimated by many.

Besides contact with hepatitis C-infected blood, how else might the virus be transmitted, and what precautions need the hepatitis C-infected individual take to prevent passing this scourge on to other people? There has been no evidence that hepatitis C has been transmitted by kissing, so routine hugging and shows of affection are not cause for alarm. One exception would be if there are open sores or wounds which might allow contact with contaminated blood. Breast milk of infected moms does not contain the virus, so the hepatitis C consensus committee feels it is reasonable to breast-feed a newborn, weighing the risks of transmission with the benefits of natural breast milk. Extreme caution must be exercised to avoid breast feeding if the nipple is raw, inflamed or denuded of its skin covering—in other words, if the nipple is prone to bleeding.

Present recommendations call for the use of a barrier contraceptive device to prevent transmission of the virus during intercourse, particularly for individuals with multiple sexual partners. Monogamous couples may choose not to use barrier contraceptives, according to CDC and NIH consensus recommendations. Though the risk of transmission is quite low, there are studies of couples who have been sexually active in monogamous relationships for many years where one individual is infected and the other is not which show a low but non-zero rate of conversion of the uninfected mate (approximately 1–3% of couples over many decades). The National Institutes of Health hepatitis C consensus committee fell short of recommending contraceptives for all monogamous couples, emphasizing the need for contraception among those with multiple sexual partners. This reluctance of the NIH hepatitis C consensus committee to take a strong stand to attempt to prevent all cases of sexually transmitted hepatitis C is controversial, and may stem from a reluctance to disrupt marital practices in order to address a very low risk of transmission. Since there seems to be a risk of transmission even in monogamous couples, it appears the use of barrier contraception will prevent a small but significant number of new cases of hepatitis C over time. Hence, it would be safest to use barrier contraceptives, preferably a condom or, less desirably, a diaphragm with spermicide for all those infected with hepatitis C and their sex partners. It should be emphasized that sexual practices that would increase the risk of transmission of blood or abrasions to mucosal surfaces would increase the risk of transmission of the virus. These practices would include unprotected intercourse at the time of the menstrual period, or unprotected rectal intercourse, either of which could place either partner at risk.

Body fluids such as stool, saliva, urine, ascitic fluid, and semen from infected individuals have been shown to contain hepatitis C RNA or minuscule trace quantities of virus at times. Transmission of the virus by these fluids is rare. All semen donated to sperm banks for artificial insemination needs to be screened for the hepatitis C virus to prevent transmission to the potential mother. While it is reassuring that these fluids do not normally contain significant quantities of the virus, it must be stressed that all of these body fluids may be contaminated with blood. Small quantities of blood in stool, breast milk, urine, saliva, or semen may not be visible to the eye but ascertained by more sensitive testing methods. To be completely safe, avoiding unnecessary contact with body fluids from an individual with hepatitis C seems prudent, particularly in settings where those fluids might come in contact with an uninfected person's blood. Blood is therefore felt to be the primary vehicle for transmission of the virus.

One of the treatments for hepatitis C, ribavirin, is a teratogen as well as being toxic to embryos. Teratogens are agents that cause malformations in developing fetuses and embryos. This can lead to the birth of offspring who have gross deformations—what are generally viewed as cataclysmic defects by new parents. Naturally, from the child's perspective this is a perfectly preventable disaster which he might have to carry with him throughout his life. People using ribavirin must be careful to use both male and female birth control during treatment and for 6 months after treatment, or their baby could be born severely deformed.

Another mode of transmission of hepatitis C is from mother to child. This route of infection is thankfully rather rare. It is estimated that probably 1 in 100 mothers infected with hepatitis C transmits the virus to her children. This is much better than some other bloodborne viruses, like HIV or hepatitis B. Another potential route of infection involves breast feeding.

Thankfully again, the evidence for transmissibility of hepatitis C from a mother to a breast-fed infant is so weak that careful breast feeding by hepatitis C-infected mothers is still acceptable practice. Care must be taken to avoid exposure to blood. As previously stated, if the mother's nipples become abraded, heavily inflamed, chapped, or grossly bloody, common sense would suggest that they be allowed to heal prior to the mother resuming breast feeding.

Healthcare workers seem to have a slightly increased risk over the general population of contracting hepatitis C. Naturally, universal precautions to avoid contact with patients' blood that were instituted in the late 1980s should be effective at mitigating exposure to hepatitis C. Hepatitis C has been around for a long time, and exposure was more likely before the use of universal precautions. Injuries in which healthcare providers are stuck with needles contaminated with infected blood are unfortunately not a rare event. That transmission by this route of inoculation is also rare is reassuring. It is much easier to transmit HIV or hepatitis B with a needlestick injury. One potentially counterintuitive note is that the administration of antibodies, gamma globulin, is not recommended if a person gets stuck with a needle contaminated with hepatitis C. The reason is that all gamma globulin is screened for antibodies to hepatitis C and units containing antibodies are discarded. Gamma globulin has therefore been deliberately manufactured to exclude antihepatitis C antibodies, so its administration to prevent hepatitis C infection would not be beneficial. New preparations of antihepatitis C antibodies are being developed.

People on dialysis also risk contracting hepatitis C. There seems to be a risk of transmission of hepatitis C during hemodialysis, when a patient with kidney failure is hooked up to a machine which performs the functions of his kidneys. It appears that the dialysis machines may be contaminated with small quantities of hepatitis C, which crosses the disposable filters designed to protect one person who uses the machine from the diseases of another. The rate of acquisition of hepatitis C is greater in people on hemodialysis than in those receiving other forms of dialysis, such as peritoneal dialysis, in which fluid is exchanged into the abdomen and a hemodialysis machine is not used.

Properly autoclaved medical equipment, such as scissors and other instruments, should not be a risk factor for transmitting hepatitis C. Similarly, dental instruments properly cleaned between uses should be safe. There is concern, though, that instruments in a barber shop or beauty shop may not be properly cleaned between customers. Often bleach, lye, or other chemical disinfectants are used to clean these instruments. If properly used, the hepatitis C virus might not survive these chemicals, though better tests of disinfectant effectiveness against this particular virus would be reassuring. The danger would increase were someone in a rush for another set of scissors or nail clippers and might not disinfect them properly. They might not, for example, soak them in the disinfectant for the normal time period or skip that step entirely. While there may be general guidelines for these establishments, they are loosely enforced, and whether these general guidelines are adequate still needs to be tested. This is an area which likely warrants government controls with health inspections similar to restaurants.

RECREATIONAL DRUGS

Rudy remembered trying heroin while in Vietnam. One day after a particularly vicious campaign in the jungle, his unit had been moved to the rear. Like vultures, the drug dealers descended on them. The whole unit shot up together. Rudy did not want to do it, but he felt that he really did not have much choice in the matter. At least it seemed that way at the time. It was the only time he had ever done anything like that, but he wondered if he could have caught hepatitis C then. He did not remember who cleaned the needles they used or whether they were cleaned at all.

Table 5.   Transmission of Hepatitis C at a Glance

Up to 20% of hepatitis C cases do not have a history of a defined high-risk exposure

Hepatitis C turns out to be the cause of 90% of the cases of transfusion-associated hepatitis before 1992

For those who use intravenous drugs and share needles, the risk of transmission is 75–90%

Transmission from a hepatitis C-infected mother to her child occurs 1–5% of the time at birth

---

The use of certain recreational drugs has been linked with hepatitis C transmission. The prevalence of recreational drug use in our society facilitates the transmission of bloodborne infections from one person to another. The greatest ongoing risk of hepatitis C transmission involves the use of intravenous drugs. Sharing of needles occurs, and therefore transmission of bloodborne viruses is common. Because the hepatitis C virus is highly prevalent in the population of the United States, the probability of transmission among IV drug users who share needles is actually fairly high, even if a needle is shared only one time with one other user. Therefore, many people who experimented with intravenous or subcutaneous drug injection during the 1960s or '70s are now testing positive for hepatitis C. Many of them may have even forgotten this simple experimentation and recall it only after careful reflection.

Another form of recreational drug use that can lead to transmission is the use of intranasal cocaine. Cocaine is an irritant to the nasal mucosa, and when it is vigorously snorted to produce a euphoric sensation it often causes mild mucosal bleeding (bloody nose). Transmission is complicated by the fact that the drug is often used in a social setting with people sharing a tooter (cocaine straw), such as a rolled-up dollar bill, which may become contaminated with small quantities of blood. In this way, the tooter or bill is inserted from one pleasure seeker's nostril into another, and blood may be transmitted from one abraded mucosal surface to another.

The use of recreational drugs and alcohol may also lead people to participate in activities they might otherwise deem dirty, unsafe or unwise. Rudy did some crazy things when he was younger, and he often worried if he might have infected some of his old friends many years ago. He often wondered how they were doing, but he had no way of getting in touch with them.

Once when Rudy was drunk several decades ago, he went under a freeway overpass with his drinking buddy Clarisse. They decided to give each other tattoos with a needle and some inks Rudy had won in a game of poker. Rudy could not remember if he gave Clarisse a tattoo first, then passed the needles to her. She wiped them off but did not sterilize them. She also dipped them into the ink that had been contaminated with blood. Rudy now wondered if Clarisse had hepatitis C and if he could have gotten the virus then. One of the problems with tracking the spread of hepatitis C infection is that the infection may come to light decades after it occurred, so the number of potential contacts may prove staggering. As in Clarisse's case, Rudy had no idea where she was currently, so he had no way of getting in touch with her. He was not even sure he remembered her name correctly.

Ironically, several decades after they exchanged tattoos, Clarisse recalled Rudy too. She was confused; she was trying to be nice and do the right thing. The Red Cross had put out a big notice about a shortage of blood, so she thought she would drop by the blood station and donate a few pints. Next thing she knew, she got a letter saying she was infected with hepatitis C. This devastated her. Here she was, just trying to help others and not look for problems, but she had a big one now. On an intellectual level, she was glad she had found out about the virus now, but emotionally she wished she had never heard of hepatitis C. Suddenly, she felt stigmatized by infection. She thought about what to do, and then threw the letter from the Red Cross in the garbage. She was too busy to deal with this now, and besides she was feeling fine. The knowledge ate away at her subconsciously as if she had committed a nasty crime she was trying to deny.

MANICURES, PEDICURES, TATTOOS, ACUPUNCTURE, AND BODY PIERCING

Hepatitis C has been associated with transmission primarily via blood transfusions or intravenous drug use and exchange of needles tainted with blood. Some studies have shown an association with tattoos, in which blood products can be transmitted from one customer to another via tattooing equipment, and other forms of person-to-person blood contamination such as body piercing. Naturally it is important not only that people be cautious when they are using such services, but also that the providers of these services be extremely careful to ensure sterility and lack of person-to-person transmission of any bloodborne infectious agents. The use of effective methods of sterilization to cleanse instruments from one person to the next is critical for insuring customer confidence in providers of these services. Some have emphasized the importance of the use of separate batches of ink, for example, in tattoo parlors.

The growing popularity of body piercing also raises the possibility of transmission during an act of piercing of tongues, eyebrows, nipples, or other body appendages—even earlobes. The facilities that provide these services are poorly regulated, and people often get pierced at home, in a college dorm, or in a shop. Since piercing is often done with friends who are amateurs in the practice or in poorly regulated centers, the problem is that blood-to-blood transmission is possible. Once again, people should exercise common sense and be particularly aware, whether they have unknown hepatitis C status or are knowingly hepatitis C-infected and intend to purchase these services, to eliminate the risk of thereby transmitting the virus to another. Piercing ears for earrings could be another source of disease transmission. Teenage girls frequently pay to have their ears pierced in shopping mall stands which may quickly disinfect their equipment with alcohol. Once again, while alcohol might destroy the virus, there is always room for doubt.

Particularly if instruments were not thoroughly soaked in alcohol one might understand how a contaminated instrument might have been used from one person to another.

Naturally, people with hepatitis C should not donate blood. While the blood supply is now checked rigorously for hepatitis C virus, people should be sure to inform any healthcare provider of hepatitis C infection and refrain from giving blood or serum. One frightening aspect of blood procurement is that companies that pay for blood are often located in indigent neighborhoods where the incidence of intravenous drug use and hepatitis C prevalence are the highest.

Acupuncture is another practice that may transmit the virus. In this medical practice of Eastern origin, needles are inserted into the body at trigger points to treat illnesses or dull pain. Since this practice is not part of mainstream Western health care, it is commonly practiced in small clinics of Eastern medicine or even out of the homes of acupuncture practitioners. At times these sites may not be equipped with autoclaves or other methods of sterilizing the needles, so the virus may be transmitted by blood-to-blood spread from one infected acupuncture client to another.

One common practice in our society is the sale of manicures and pedicures at commercial beauty saloons to enhance appearance. Once again, instruments such as probes, nail clippers and scissors are used to trim nails, and these may be contaminated with blood. Similarly, nail polish, nail polish remover, and fillers all might also come to be contaminated with blood if someone bleeds during a beauty-enhancing session. It is difficult to determine exactly whether these might transmit the virus if contaminated with tainted blood, but in the absence of hard scientific data, concern is appropriate. If two people have open wounds on their hands or around their nails, the risk of blood-to-blood transmission of virus exists. Similarly, if a beautician, either amateur or professional, is overly aggressive in trimming or manicuring nails, bleeding may ensue. Even small amounts of bleeding may be sufficient to transmit the virus. It would seem prudent for the providers of beauty services to be better regulated and inspected by the health department to ensure sterile techniques which eliminate the risk of virus transmission. Certainly any individual purchasing a manicure or pedicure or sharing instruments with friends is taking a risk unless using an autoclave on all instruments to avoid person-to-person transmission of any bloodborne pathogens. Since it is hard to define exactly what constitutes a safe sterilization procedure and ensure that it is properly followed, perhaps cautious manicure patrons could bring their own metal tools, nail polish remover, emery board, buffer, filler, nail polish, etc.

Barber shops create another potential environment for blood-to-blood transmission. Scissors, razors, combs, brushes, and electric razors all pose a risk for becoming contaminated with blood. There is broad variation in cleanliness from one barber shop to another. Some are quite filthy, with instruments sterilized briefly if at all between one patron and another. Similarly, just as cases of HIV have been documented to have been transmitted at dentist's offices which did not practice appropriate sterile techniques, hepatitis C may have well been transferred at the time of dental procedures as well.

While blood-to-blood transmission would be an admittedly rare event by these routes, the approximately 20% of people infected with chronic hepatitis C who do not have a risk factor for transmission suggests that there may be common practices in society that can transmit the virus. This uncertainty leads to speculation as to what these practices may in fact be. Alternatively, because the transmission may have occurred decades before diagnosis, some of these people who do not have risk factors may just lack the memory of an elephant and actually have caught hepatitis C while engaging in one of the known risk factors for transmission.

Some may wonder if mosquitoes are a vector for transmitting hepatitis C. After all, mosquitoes bite one person, sucking up their blood, and then bite another. Malaria is a common infection transmitted by mosquitoes. While it is difficult to exclude the possibility that someone stung by a thousand mos-

Table 6. Recommendations to Reduce Transmission

Health care workers follow universal precautions; assume everyone is infected

Hepatitis C-infected individuals should not donate blood, semen, organs, or tissues

People who have used intravenous recreational drugs or snorted cocaine should not donate blood

Barrier methods of contraception, particularly for people with more than one partner. Test sexual partners of hepatitis C-infected people to determine if they have caught the virus

Decrease household transmission

Test babies born to HCV-positive mothers at 1 year of age

Consider needle exchange programs or other measures to prevent transmission among people who indulge in intravenous drugs

Educate people to prevent transmission

Develop and distribute a safe and effective vaccine

---

quitoes with hepatitis C in their system might not catch the disease, the best statistical evidence for transmission shows no increased risk of transmission in areas with lots of mosquitoes in comparison to those with few. The best present evidence suggests that people should not worry about mosquito bites as a way of catching hepatitis C.

Thank goodness the rate of transmission of hepatitis C between infected individuals and their family members is quite low. It is suspected that transmission does infrequently occur, and once again may come from sources of blood-to-blood transmission such as shared toothbrushes, razors, or kitchen utensils, particularly in the setting of poor dental hygiene or bleeding gums. People who live closely together also are more likely to be exposed to each other's blood. Young children playing may bite each other. As in Mark Twain's novel, some people may deliberately mix their blood, fancying themselves brazen, like Huck Finn. When people cut themselves and are bleeding, a loved one's first reaction is to help them. This may lead to exposure to infected blood as well. Direct blood contact at the time of injury should be stringently avoided by household contacts of hepatitis C-infected individuals. If someone with hepatitis C is cut and bleeds on the kitchen counter, they should tend to their wound themselves if possible or seek professional help. Thinking ahead, family members might want to have protective rubber gloves handy so that they can help a relative in case of an accident in which hepatitis C-infected blood was exposed. If at all possible, hepatitis C-infected individuals should clean up their blood themselves using bleach and not allow anyone else to be exposed to it. Since it is rather difficult to transmit hepatitis C, there is no evidence to justify excluding infected people from jobs, school, or social activities. People infected with hepatitis C should not become the victims of discrimination as well.

Fortunately, the number of new transmissions of hepatitis C is less this year than it was 10 years ago. The virus is easily transmitted by blood-to-blood exposure, but appears to be harder to transmit by other routes. Careful measures to screen our blood supply and exclude units tainted with hepatitis C as well as safer sex and safer recreational drug habits are having an impact. One question that remains is how a rather large fraction (up to 20%) of infected people caught the virus without a clear history of "high-risk" blood exposure. Perhaps even more care needs to be taken to prevent blood-to-blood transmission at barber shops and beauty parlors. Certainly, more aggressive measures to stem transmission start with identifying those already infected so that they may practice the utmost care to prevent their blood from exposing others. The development of a safe and effective vaccine will be another milestone in efforts to prevent new cases of infection.

7

Hepatitis C and Alcohol

Another area which warrants special comment is the interaction between hepatitis C and alcohol. This is a particularly difficult area to discuss because of the varied levels of consumption of alcohol and the fact that many people who drink alcohol are in a state of denial. Suffice it to say that many people have realized that if they use alcohol, even in moderation, they may develop a fairly severe liver disease if they are infected with hepatitis C. They may notice others around them drinking similar quantities of alcohol without serious consequences. It is not uncommon for people with liver disease to say such things as, "Gee, my friend Ralph drinks twice as much as I do, and he doesn't have any liver problems."

The "safe" level of alcohol use is difficult to identify because it is quite variable from one individual to another. People have grappled with this dilemma. We have seen many patients with hepatitis C who drink one or two drinks a day, a combination that can contribute to a fairly severe case of liver disease. It is therefore prudent to eliminate routine consumption of alcohol if infected with hepatitis C, because there is mounting evidence demonstrating that there is no safe level of alcohol consumption for the hepatitis C-infected person. While some physicians counsel their patients that it is safe to drink several drinks a day, recent clinical studies do not support this casual attitude. In contrast, it is my opinion that in the absence of good epidemiologic data demonstrating the safety of this amount of alcohol given hepatitis C, it is wise to avoid it entirely.

Dr. Bates reminded Rudy that alcohol affects not only his mood, but also his body and the medicines he takes. Alcohol acts like other mood-altering drugs in the body, with its primary desired effects on the brain and nervous system. Alcohol also can cause inflammation or bleeding in the stomach, inflammation of the pancreas, and inflammation or ultimate scarring of the liver. The severity of the effects of alcohol is influenced by the drinker's genetic background, current state of health, and level of consumption.

The United States government tried to ban alcohol in the early 1900s, mainly because of the efforts of temperance activists who blamed the drug for physical illnesses and moral dissipation. The desire for alcohol was so great, though, that the attempt at prohibition brought an era of bootlegging and related crimes, and formerly law-abiding citizens became patrons of illicit speakeasies. Today only children's access to alcohol is restricted—among other reasons, because of its powerful toxicity to the developing nervous system. The government now warns pregnant women not to consume alcohol because its use can lead to underweight, maldeveloped infants with fetal alcohol syndrome. Despite extensive warnings and concerns, the majority of American adults still consume alcohol.

Dr. Bates put his hand on Rudy's shoulder and explained, "Rudy, it is important to remember that alcohol affects different people differently." Even more important, Dr. Bates continued, it is critical that you understand that alcohol can affect the same person differently at different times. How healthy your liver is can have a tremendous impact on how liquor affects you. Similarly, if you have not drunk in a long time, alcohol can build up more quickly in your system than if you were drinking regularly. How much you weigh and whether you are drinking with food or on an empty stomach can also affect how much alcohol you can drink before becoming drunk.

Alcohol's primary action is as a central nervous system depressant, much like benzodiazepines such as Valium. Rudy was half-listening to Bates's lecture at this point. Silently, he sang to himself the phrase to the Ramones song, "I want to be sedated, bam, bam, ba-bam, bam, ba-bam, bam, ba-bam, I want to be sedated." Bates continued on, explaining that small quantities of alcohol relax inhibitions opening us up to risky behavior. Alcohol can also dissolve the cells lining the food pipe, or esophagus, and stomach. This can lead to inflammation of the stomach or gastritis and bleeding. While the effects of a moderate amount of alcohol consumption on the stomach and esophagus are usually reversible if you stop drinking alcohol, more intense consumption can lead to recurrent damage and scar formation.

Alcohol is normally broken down in the liver prior to its elimination from the body. Chronic alcohol use can lead to serious complications in the liver. People used to think that *excessive* consumption was necessary to cause severe damage to the liver. Now we know that certain people with a susceptible genetic makeup may be more prone than others to liver injury from alcohol. Just like blond hair, blue eyes or big noses can run in families, increased susceptibility to alcohol-induced liver damage can run in families too.

There also is synergy between alcohol and hepatitis C in causing liver damage. Since the liver is the organ that processes alcohol, as the liver gets sicker, alcohol may accumulate for longer periods of time and to higher levels in the body. Alcohol consumption may lead to inflammation of the liver, which is characterized by a chronic elevation of liver enzymes leaking into the blood, and in more severe forms may manifest as alcoholic hepatitis. This is a form of hepatitis caused by ingesting a toxin, alcohol, as opposed to catching an infection like viral hepatitis. During acute alcoholic hepatitis, the liver becomes painful and swollen, which leads to decreased function and jaundice. The end point of chronic inflammation is the formation of scar tissue in the liver, or fibrosis. Once this scarring has progressed in the liver, it is termed cirrhosis.

Alcohol consumption can affect medicines, both over-the-counter and prescription. How does it affect them? Alcohol can alter the metabolism or rate of elimination of over 100 medicines from the body. Alcohol can interact with a medicine to make it toxic even at the recommended doses for a sober person. Dangerous interactions between alcohol and other drugs have occurred both with transient acute alcohol use and with chronic alcohol use. Similarly, bad reactions to medicines may accumulate over time, or they may be quite temporary and acute.

Alcohol–drug interaction warnings are included with many over-the-counter pain relievers like Tylenol, Motrin, and Naproxen. What is all the fuss about? Tylenol, or acetaminophen, can cause severe liver injury when taken in excessive doses. Nevertheless, when Tylenol is taken by people who chronically drink several drinks a day, the dose necessary to cause severe liver injury is less than in a sober person. Chronic heavy alcohol drinkers are therefore at increased risk for Tylenol-induced liver injury. It is therefore particularly important that individuals who drink large amounts of alcohol pay careful attention not to exceed the recommended doses of Tylenol. Since alcohol can irritate the stomach, interactions with nonsteroidal anti-inflammatory drugs, or NSAIDs, like aspirin, Motrin, and Naproxen can lead to an increased risk for GI bleeding. Since alcohol is a sedative, it may also interact with other sedatives like Benadryl or barbiturates to produce excessive drowsiness or increased sedation. While these effects are dose dependent, or related to the quantity of alcohol or sedative used, the degree of sedation may be synergistic, or greater than the amount of sedation one would expect from merely adding the sedative properties of the one agent to those of the other. Narcotic pain medicines like codeine or Percocet can lead to greater confusion and drowsiness when taken with alcohol. Antidepressants that are so prevalent in society like Prozac, Elavil, and MAO inhibitors can cause greater sedative effects, drowsiness, confusion and other CNS effects. Alcohol can interact with oral antidiabetics like Micronase to cause altered blood sugar control, such as more frequent hypo-glycemia or low blood sugars. Alcohol can also interact with the common antibiotic flagyl to produce facial flushing, head-ache, nausea, vomiting, and abdominal distress.

Rudy came back to reality as Dr. Bates finished his solilo-quy. He now realized that alcohol could cause problems even in moderate doses. The toxic effects of alcohol on the liver are synergistic with the bad effects of hepatitis C infection. Rudy also understood that many common prescription and over-the-counter drugs interact with alcohol, and that he needed to be careful to take his medicines as prescribed, and to avoid ex-ceeding the recommended doses for over-the-counter medi-cines. Most importantly, since he was infected with hepatitis C, Rudy faced the fact that he needed to stop drinking com-pletely.

8

The Search for the Holy Grail

Universally effective treatments for hepatitis C have eluded researchers so far. The most common treatment is interferon therapy, which boosts the body's own immune system to fight off the virus. Experimental protocols have established that prolonging the length of treatment from 6 months to 1 year increases the percentage of people who respond favorably to treatment. Other current experimental trials remove some iron from serum to lower iron levels in the body by means of bleeding therapy before or during interferon therapy. The idea is that iron might interfere with the action of interferon or boost the damage caused by the virus. Data to demonstrate which patients may benefit are still being collected. Still other clinical studies have used interferon in combination with other drugs, and these trials have netted some successes as well as some failures. The combination of interferon and ribavirin (a second antiviral drug) looks particularly promising and has been approved by the FDA, but still, fewer than half of the infected individuals treated with this combination have been

cured in experimental protocols. The combination of interferon and amantidine (another antiviral drug), which seemed
to be a miracle several years ago after tiny clinical trials
showed promise, now does not show much promise after careful study. It is important to remember, too, that experimental
protocols study a highly select group of individuals. These
protocol patients are preselected to be highly motivated and
compliant with the treatment regimens. They also do not have
other coexisting diseases, such as alcoholism or diabetes,
which might influence response to treatment. The majority of
people in the general population do not have hepatitis C as
their only medical problem. Often, people with infection complicated by cirrhosis or decompensated cirrhosis may be excluded from these protocols. For this reason, the response
rates to medications in a highly select group of individuals
enrolled in a protocol may be higher than the response rate in
the general population. Several studies of nonselected patient
populations provide evidence to support a lower response rate
in the general population.

There certainly are many exciting new treatments on the
horizon. The fact that interferon works at all is truly a miracle.
In comparison to HIV, against which drugs inhibiting viral
replication (viral protease inhibitors) prolong the carrier's survival but do not actually cure the infection, hepatitis C infection can be cured (albeit in only a small proportion, perhaps
10–20% of those infected), which is cause for some hope and
optimism.

Hepatitis C also has nonstructural proteins which help the
virus to replicate inside of the cells. These would be like the
weapons carried inside the belly of the Trojan horse. These
weapons are essential for the virus to function, copy itself and
make more virus. For example, one of these molecules cleaves
long viral proteins, which do not function themselves, into
several smaller, working ones. It is called a viral protease. It's
as if several bikes are chained together, and they need to
be unlocked before they can be ridden. Specific molecules
called trypsin inhibitors may be made to inhibit viral protease

function—that is, inhibit the molecules that unlock viral protein function. Trypsin inhibitors work as if someone squirted Krazy Glue into a door lock; even if you have a key, you cannot unlock the lock. Certainly the HIV protease inhibitors are the most common form of clinically available medicines that act through this blocking mechanism. Unfortunately, since HIV and hepatitis C have different molecules, it does not appear that the HIV inhibitors are active against hepatitis C.

HIV protease inhibitors represent a milestone in therapy for HIV, greatly prolonging the life of infected people. The introduction of HIV protease inhibitors brought about a dramatic improvement in the well-being of individuals infected with HIV. The HIV protease inhibitors are able to decrease the amount of HIV virus in the blood 100-fold to 1000-fold. As many people are aware, HIV is now often treated with a cocktail, or mixture of drugs. Since they work so well, the center piece of these cocktails is a protease inhibitor, with names such as Saquinavir, Indinavir, and Ritonavir. The addition of two other drugs active against HIV from another class of antiviral compounds (nucleoside analogs like lamividine and AZT) reduces the amount of virus in the blood another 10-fold. People are obviously excited about developing similar approaches to treat hepatitis C.

How long will it be before we have protease inhibitors available for therapy that cripple the hepatitis C virus? HIV protease inhibitors were designed or engineered by deducing a three-dimensional structure of the HIV protease "lock" and then engineering "keys" which fit in the lock cylinder, filling it and blocking the lock from turning, blocking the protease from making functional HIV proteins. The HIV lock structure (protease crystals) was deduced in 1988, and it took 8 years before HIV protease inhibitors came to market after this first step. The hepatitis C protease (lock) was crystallized in 1996. If we use the development of inhibitor treatments for HIV as a barometer, one would hope that by the year 2004 specific small molecules that inhibit the hepatitis C viral protease will be available on the market.

Who funds the research for treatments of hepatitis C? Is enough being done to find more effective treatments? Is a cure likely? The answers to these questions are somewhat complicated. The state of liver research in this country is quite good, but it could be better. The National Institutes of Health (NIH) devotes only a small fraction of its budget to studying all liver diseases. But the liver makes up 12% of the body, and 2% of the U.S. population is infected with hepatitis C. The reason, like most things in Washington, involves politics. The NIH is divided into individual institutes, such as the National Heart, Lung and Blood Institute; the National Institute of Mental Health; the National Institute of Allergy and Infectious Diseases; and the National Institute of Diabetes, Digestive and Kidney Diseases. Money flows into the NIH from Congress and the president as part of the federal budget. It is then doled out to individual institutes, which operate almost like medieval fiefdoms. They spend about 12% of the budget for research on intramural programs on the NIH campus in Bethesda, Maryland. The remainder of the money is sent to predominantly academic medical centers around the country in the form of peer-reviewed grants. Within the diabetes, digestive and kidney disease institute, what fraction goes to liver diseases? Historically, it has not been as much as people with liver disease would like. Diabetes research needs to be well funded; there are outstanding lobbies advocating its support, and a large research infrastructure has been established which needs to be supported. Kidney diseases have also attracted a large share of support. Liver diseases are supported through a portion of the digestive disease budget, which includes diseases of seven organs in the body: esophagus, stomach, small intestine, large intestine, pancreas, gallbladder, and liver. Similarly, diseases like cancer and HIV have strong lobbies or advocates that extol the virtues of funding research in their prospective areas. While funding any biomedical research is laudable, liver diseases deserve their fair share of the research funding pie. The National Institutes of Health is recognizing the importance of hepatitis C research and is now greatly increasing the funds available for research in this area.

As recently as 50 years ago, not much was known about how the liver worked, so we lacked effective treatments for liver disease. Since it was not easy to obtain liver samples for study, liver research initially lagged behind other areas of research, such as hematology or oncology. As these areas developed, they commanded larger portions of the NIH budget. There also was a stigma attached to liver diseases as society cynically views liver disease as the patient's own fault: excessive alcohol consumption.

This bias against people with liver disease is unfortunate, unfair, and in many cases undeserved. Housewives, lawyers, doctors, nurses, teachers, business people, and factory workers all get liver diseases, and many of them drink little or no alcohol. What is very interesting is the cultural difference in the United States between the way liver disease and cardiac disease are approached. People with liver disease are often blamed for bringing this fate upon themselves through excessive consumption of alcohol. People with heart disease, who may have precipitated their illness with consumption of a high-fat diet and smoking, are often treated more sympathetically. They are more open about telling family and friends about their illness, and their illnesses receive more support from the federal government for research. Perhaps the bias against people with liver disease is one of the last vestiges of the failed attempt at alcohol prohibition in the beginning of this century. This contrasts with other societies, such as France, where liver disease is much more socially accepted. If someone in France feels weak or not otherwise well, it is not uncommon for them to rub the area over their liver and proclaim that their liver must be sick. This ascribing the symptoms of an illnesses to poor liver health is much like someone in this country singling out his headache as the symptom of his illness, and holding his hand to his forehead. The open acceptance of people with liver disease certainly facilitates individuals coping with their illness, and it is important that our society overcome any cultural stigmas associated with liver disease if liver research is to advance at a maximal possible pace.

There was a small club of liver doctors who formed an

organization known as the AASLD, or American Association for the Study of Liver Diseases, 50 years ago in Chicago. This group has since met on an annual basis to exchange ideas and share their progress in liver research and clinical hepatology. Up until the 1970s, this organization was a rather exclusive club with a small membership. As members of this group discussed each others' studies, in the 1970s their research was relatively well funded even as liver diseases in general were shunned for federal funding relative to cancer, heart disease, and diabetes. Recognizing the importance of lobbying the government for research support, the AASLD spun off a subsidiary organization to lobby for issues related to liver diseases and to raise funds for liver research, the American Liver Foundation (ALF). This organization has also established itself as a cutting-edge patient educator, with national campaigns such as the "yellow eyes" campaign to educate the public about hepatitis and liver diseases. One reason the ALF was spun off from the AASLD was to permit the raising of funds from industry without the potential conflicts of interest which might be present if the AASLD were involved in soliciting funds from pharmaceutical companies. Nevertheless, the AASLD has participated in lobbying and fund raising over time. Several more recent organizations have formed to address similar fund raising, patient education and lobbying concerns, such as the Hepatitis Foundation International, and more recently the highly successful American Digestive Health Foundation.

Over the last three decades, the AASLD has made a vigorous effort to welcome new members and has grown into the premier international liver society. The organization has outrun its usual meeting quarters in Chicago, and annual meetings will be held in locations which may change from one year to the next, starting in 1999. The AASLD also started the journal *Hepatology* 30 years ago. While this is the most prestigious journal of liver medicine in this country, it contains an eclectic blend of clinical and basic science research. It is surprising that some of the best basic research in liver diseases is performed by scientists with no formal training in hepatology and published in basic science journals which are seldom read by clinical hepatologists.

So if the government has not invested heavily in hepatitis C research, and there is not a large cadre of talented liver doctors doing basic research on hepatitis C, what is fueling discovery in the field of hepatitis C research? Our market-based economy has compelled companies to work on hepatitis C, and they have responded impressively. Scientists at Chiron, as mentioned previously, discovered the virus and developed diagnostic kits to screen blood and assist in identifying infected individuals. The major pharmaceutical companies Schering-Plough, Amgen, and Roche Pharmaceuticals have developed immunotherapies for hepatitis C. The costs of the clinical trials necessary to bring these drugs to market can exceed $200 million. The cost of some single trials has exceeded $60 million. Along with these huge costs come high prices for interferon treatment. A 1-year course of interferon costs thousands of dollars.

So is there a problem with companies driving the lion's share of research in hepatitis C? Developing new treatments takes time, money, skill, and luck. One of the companies best situated to develop treatments for hepatitis C, Chiron, is in the process of developing treatments to bring to market. There are several disadvantages to relying strictly on companies to develop treatments for hepatitis C. First, companies may be restricted in what they are willing to discuss publicly. In other words, information at two different companies may be at the very least duplicative and at the worst essential for further discovery only if shared. Companies can easily work only on treatments for which they hold patents or for which they may acquire patents in the future. Cross-licensing agreements to share technology are possible when scientists and business people from different companies cooperate. If some discoveries are kept secret, mutually beneficial relationships may not become obvious. In short, companies do not want to bolster a competitor's patent position or develop a treatment that virtually anyone can market at profit. This restricts the scope of potential treatments companies may work on. Finally, companies may exhaust great resources, patients' time, and clinical investigators' time on treatments which in the end may provide only an incremental improvement. There is a great deal of futile activity involved in cutting-edge discovery. Collaborations among university investigators, research institute investigators, and pharmaceutical companies hold the greatest promise of advancing our treatments for hepatitis C as rapidly as possible.

Clearly, the field of hepatitis C research could benefit greatly from the application of the technologies that have so greatly assisted the search for a cure for HIV. There is a pressing need for the establishment of hepatitis C institutes dedicated to studying the virus, and the National Institutes of Health is responding to public concerns by developing focused grant programs to address the problems of hepatitis C. Investigation into the epidemiology, virology, and natural course of hepatitis C infection is entering an era of logarithmic growth, leading to leaps in new knowledge. Now that we are gaining this new knowledge, it can only fuel further discoveries as time passes.

There is growing optimism that hepatitis C research is beginning to receive the attention that so many infected people and their families feel it deserves. Meaningful physician education initiatives are now under way to promote increased knowledge of hepatitis C infection and its consequences. Multiple media outlets, such as the Internet, television, tapes, CD interactive learning programs, journals, and books, are all leading to the rapid dissemination of the information about hepatitis C throughout society. As infected people demand greater research initiatives in hepatitis C, Congress and the NIH are responding by setting aside funds earmarked for hepatitis C research. Liver societies such as the AASLD, ADHF, and ALF have all successfully lobbied for increased research funding on behalf of member physicians and their patients.

Rapid advances are being made in hepatitis C research by both academic investigators and corporations with vested interests. There is considerable collaboration among various groups to study the natural history of infection and develop new treatment regimens. There is a growing swell of support for greater investment in hepatitis C research, and this is occurring as a broader appreciation of the magnitude of the disease is developing. Early successes such as interferon therapy have cured a fraction of the patients infected with hepatitis C and have raised the hopes of millions of infected individuals that they, too, may one day be cured as new treatments are developed.

9

Diet and Nutrition

Since chronic hepatitis C infection progresses to cirrhotic liver disease from several years to many decades after infection, one obvious question is how to delay or prevent this progression. Treating the virus to eliminate it is one good idea, but this is not successful in the majority of cases. Exactly what determines who progresses slowly and who progresses rapidly is not completely understood. *Perhaps the single most important measure anyone infected with hepatitis C may take to slow disease progression is to avoid alcohol.*

Diet certainly may be a factor affecting the rate of disease progression, as diet influences the immune system, influences our overall state of well-being and plays an important role in the pathogenesis of other diseases, such as coronary artery disease. We know far less about the impact of diet on liver diseases than, for example, the role cholesterol plays in atherosclerotic coronary artery disease—heart disease. When Dr. Bates rotated through the coronary care unit, he was struck by the number of people with acute heart attacks who rolled through the doors on gurneys. The vast majority of these heart attacks could have been prevented by eliminating animal fats from the diet, lowering cholesterol, and exercise. He decided to become a vegetarian.

The guidelines for a good diet for your liver are not clear and do not have large individual outcome studies, like the Framingham Heart Study, to support specific dietary recommendations. In the absence of these clear scientific directives, common sense should reign. The diet should provide the right amount of calories to maintain an ideal nutritional state. Maintaining a healthy diet may help the liver regenerate itself or grow new liver cells. Breakdown products of most of the food substances we eat and drink pass from the bowel into the portal blood vessels and course through the liver. Balance in the diet is essential; too much of everything is not just enough. Most Americans eat too much fat in their diet, so a lower-fat diet seems prudent unless severe weight loss is a problem. Diets that use more carbohydrates as a fuel source may prove superior to those that rely too heavily on fats or protein as a source of energy, as excess dietary fats in particular can be difficult to digest and lead to obesity.

Liver disease can lead to fatigue, weight loss, and muscle wasting, particularly in the large arm and leg muscles closest to the trunk of the body. In its end stages, liver disease can grossly disfigure a person's appearance and alter their body image. As Clarisse got sicker, she found herself fawning in front of the mirror. She had once been quite attractive, and she longed for her old image which had so quickly deteriorated as her liver failed. As she went to the liver clinic, she noticed that the other people with end-stage liver disease frequently appeared old or weathered, as if they had lived a hard life. Talking to them in the waiting room, she was surprised to learn how young many of them were in terms of their actual biologic age; she would have guessed they were much older. She mentioned to Dr. Bates that her appetite was no damn good. He reassured her that this was a complaint common to many patients with end-stage liver disease, and that she might try spreading out multiple small meals throughout the day to maintain her weight.

Clarisse noticed her skin becoming drier and covered with scales as her liver failed. Clarisse's skin also started to itch interminably. This discomfort kept her awake at night at times. The difficulty sleeping made her even more tired during the day. She did not want to take any sleeping medicines as these might build up in her body owing to the inability of her failing liver to rid her body of both natural and medicinal waste products.

She had never paid much attention to the food she ate. She just ate whatever she felt like eating, but as her liver failed Clarisse became particularly interested in the effects of diet on the progression of her liver disease. She hated going to the doctor and seeing so many sick people in the waiting room. She did not want to become like the worst of them.

So what can be done to treat your liver right in terms of nutrition? The answer depends in part on the severity of the liver disease at the time the question is asked. In other words, dietary recommendations vary depending on the degree of liver dysfunction someone is experiencing.

In the early stages of hepatitis C infection, the most important dietary modification is to avoid toxins that might further damage the liver. These would include excessive doses of Tylenol or other drugs known to be hepatotoxic, as well as environmental toxins such as industrial chemicals known to injure the liver. Maintaining a balanced caloric intake and avoiding excessive obesity are prudent as well. Moderate exercise under the supervision of a physician and a reasonable amount of time for rest each day make good sense.

Just as fat is distributed throughout the body as one gains extra weight, the liver is not a sacred space spared the deposition of fat cells. In fact, overweight people frequently suffer from a "fatty liver," or liver infiltrated with fat cells. Fatty infiltration may be suggested by ultrasound or CT scan imaging studies, but it is only definitively diagnosed with a liver biopsy. Generally this excess fat sits quietly in the liver, as it does in other parts of the body. On occasion, the fatty infiltration can be associated with inflammation, or "steatohepatitis."

When this occurs, the inflammation associated with some cases of fatty infiltration of the liver can lead to cirrhosis. This kind of fatty infiltration of the liver is more common in individuals with diabetes. Alcohol use may also lead to fatty infiltration of the liver accompanied by inflammation. Fatty liver and steatohepatitis may be suggested by imaging studies but are usually diagnosed by liver biopsy. Treatments include careful weight control and control of contributing factors such as diabetes. People suffering with diabetes should attempt outstanding diabetic control through a low-sugar diet and appropriate medications if necessary.

Losing weight is never easy, but patients with hepatitis C infection and obesity should consider adhering to a low-fat, weight-reducing diet accompanied by exercise. The most reliable way to lose weight is to eat a well-balanced diet with fewer calories than you have been eating to reduce fat stores. One encouraging note is that as patients with fatty infiltration of the liver lose weight, their serum liver enzymes generally improve.

In the earlier stages of liver disease, patients with elevated triglyceride levels in the blood, hypertriglyceridemia, should follow a low cholesterol diet. High triglycerides may lead to increases in fat deposition in the liver. By keeping serum triglyceride levels within the normal range, individuals may reduce the risk of fat buildup in the liver.

Cholesterol is made and processed in the liver. As liver disease progresses, cholesterol levels may actually fall as the liver loses its ability to normally handle cholesterol. Patients with end-stage liver disease seldom have to obsess with the cholesterol content of their diet for this reason.

The prothrombin time is a measure of the amount of time it takes a sample of blood to clot. The clotting factors which allow the blood to clot are manufactured in the liver, so as the ability of the liver to make clotting factors is compromised in end-stage liver disease, the prothrombin time goes up. Several of the clotting factors made in the liver which contribute to the prothrombin time require absorption of dietary vitamin K for their production.

One objective of a healthy nutrition program for hepatitis C-induced liver disease is to prevent vitamin and mineral deficiencies or excesses. In end-stage liver disease, as bilirubin levels rise, the body may have difficulty absorbing the so-called fat-soluble vitamins, specifically vitamins A, D, E, and K. Up to 20% of patients with liver disease may have deficiencies of these vitamins. Such difficulties can lead to a prolongation of the prothrombin time due to a nutritional deficiency of vitamin K. Patients who have hepatitis C and who abuse alcohol may develop malabsorption of these vitamins on the basis of alcohol-induced injury of the pancreas. Similarly, two rare liver diseases people with hepatitis C might coincidentally also have, primary biliary cirrhosis and primary sclerosing cholangitis, can also make the absorption of the fat-soluble vitamins difficult. People who are eating poorly or not eating a well-balanced diet from the various food groups should generally take a multivitamin (it is important to check with your physician to see if this should or should not contain iron). In someone who has used a considerable amount of alcohol or developed alcoholic liver disease, thiamine and folic acid may be depleted.

In cases of severe cholestasis, when the bilirubin level gets really high, oral supplementation of fat-soluble vitamins may prove inadequate to correct the vitamin deficiency. This is because the fat-soluble vitamins when taken as pills are not easily absorbed in the setting of markedly elevated bilirubin levels. Sometimes it is necessary to supplement vitamin K with subcutaneous or intramuscular injections in the setting of severe jaundice. This obviously needs to be done at the direction of a physician.

People with end-stage liver disease may be troubled by excess fluid retention, ascites, or fluid collecting in the abdomen, and fluid collecting around the ankles. People who suffer from fluid retention are frequently treated with medicines and asked to adhere to a salt and fluid restriction. This can be difficult to do, as has been outlined elsewhere, in the section on end-stage liver disease.

Patients with end-stage liver disease also frequently develop difficulty regulating their blood sugars. The liver responds to insulin levels in the blood either to take up sugar and store its energy in the form of glycogen or to break down glycogen and release sugar into the blood. This helps to keep blood sugar levels relatively constant regardless of meals or energy demands. If the liver is sick, glycogen stores may be depleted and alternative sources of energy, such as muscle and fat, may be tapped between meals. To prevent long periods of fasting and the frequent occurrence of bouts of hypoglycemia in the patient with severe liver disease, a regimen of numerous small, frequent meals is often used to keep sugar levels in the serum more constant.

Perhaps no nutritional topic evokes more controversy than the proper amount of protein in the diet of the patient with liver disease. Protein is a key energy source, and it is essential that some of the amino acids be obtained in the diet for life. Proteins carry out critical functions throughout our body. There is a debate among nutritional experts as to how much protein people with liver disease and encephalopathy (confusion) should be eating.

The liver processes proteins, degrading their building blocks, or amino acids, to rid the body of unneeded excesses. The liver also tinkers with these molecular building blocks to rearrange them into new proteins which the body needs. Sufficient dietary protein is therefore needed to build and maintain muscles as the body breaks down muscle mass to use it as a source of energy if dietary and hepatic synthetic sources cannot keep up with the body's needs. The breakdown of muscle, which results in a gaunt, wasted appearance, is a bad sign for patients with end-stage liver disease. People with end-stage liver disease and muscle wasting tend to fair poorer with liver transplantation; perhaps they just don't have the energy reserves to deal with the stresses of the operation. People who are burning up their muscles as a source of energy obviously become weaker and are also more prone to infection. Maintaining an adequate diet can help improve liver function by providing the liver with the fuel it needs to build proteins. It may also provide the liver cells the energy they need to divide and repopulate the liver.

While guidelines vary, daily consumption of 1 to 1.5 grams of protein per kilogram (1 kilogram is 2.2 pounds) body weight is a general guideline for an otherwise healthy, nonobese person with liver disease. In other words, the amount of protein one should ingest depends on an individual's body weight. Protein consumption may be reduced in the setting of other medical diseases, such as obesity and kidney disease, so diets should be worked out under the care of a physician.

Some patients with scarring over of the liver, or cirrhosis, develop confusion, or encephalopathy. This confusion is very loosely correlated with the buildup of protein breakdown products in the blood which the liver normally processes. Why some people get encephalopathy and others don't is a question nutritional scientists are in the process of figuring out. The precise mechanism of encephalopathy is similarly being studied. Up until the time encephalopathy sets in, it is prudent to maintain adequate protein levels in the diet as a source of energy. While some physicians counsel their patients to maintain dietary protein intake even in face of substantial confusion, others disagree. They suggest limiting dietary protein to 0.6 to 0.8 grams per day of animal-derived protein or even following a vegetarian diet. There are over 20 amino acids, and proteins derived from vegetables tend to contain fewer of the specific types of amino acids that may make confusion worse than proteins derived from animals or meats. Strict vegetable diets may not contain a proper balance of amino acids to keep up weight and strength, however. When nonobese people reach end-stage liver disease, they are generally encouraged to eat as much protein as they can without succumbing to hepatic encephalopathy or confusion.

Large amounts of protein in the diet can lead to the

buildup of protein breakdown products in the blood which are normally eliminated through the liver. As this becomes too severe, it seems confusion may ensue. When we break down protein, one of the substances we make from it is called ammonia. This ammonia can circulate in the blood, and as it passes through the liver the ammonia is in turn converted to another breakdown product, urea. While urea is easily gotten rid of in the urine, ammonia builds up in the blood if the damaged liver is not able to properly convert it. There is a loose correlation between serum ammonia levels and confusion. Some physicians check ammonia levels, but this is a difficult test for laboratories to run precisely and it is therefore an inexact measure of the degree of confusion. Many physicians do not find checking ammonia levels helpful. In the patient with hepatic encephalopathy, there are also loose correlations between serum ammonia levels and the amount of protein taken in the diet.

Some people with encephalopathy seem to be more sensitive than others to protein in the diet. In other words, not everyone with encephalopathy is the same. Some may eat large quantities of dietary protein without developing any obvious change in their symptoms, while others will eat just a little bit extra protein and become quite confused. It seems that tailoring protein restrictions to the individual is the prudent approach.

Protein is available in the diet from a broad range of food sources. It is best to maintain a balanced source of protein in the diet from a variety of food sources. This is to insure that the broad range of amino acids is ingested. Fat does not contain any protein, so consumption of cooking oils, butter or animal fat does not contribute to meeting a person's dietary protein needs. Fruit, while an excellent source of fiber, also contains very little protein. Vegetables are lower in protein than meats or dairy goods, which are relatively high in protein. Ultimately, the protein content of a healthy diet is best tailored to an individual's dietary objectives and medical needs.

Table 7. Protein Content of Common Foods

Milk	8 grams/cup
Beef, chicken, fish, eggs, cheese	7 grams/1 ounce
Pasta, rice	6 grams/cup
Bread	3 grams/slice
Vegetables	4 grams/cup

Dietary iron may also play a role in the rate with which hepatitis C progresses. Although we do not fully understand why, patients with hepatitis C are often noted to have increased iron levels in their body. The liver is the main site of iron storage in the body, and perhaps the ongoing infection of the liver disrupts normal regulation of iron levels.

Regulation of the amount of iron in the body is important. Iron is a fairly toxic compound to living cells when it is present in excess. We absorb about 1–2 mg iron a day in our diet. Much of the iron is bound to special iron-mobilizing proteins, or transferrins. Iron is critical for the function of many important molecules in the body, including hemoglobin, which transports oxygen in the blood. If we have too little oxygen, we become anemic and some of our proteins won't work quite optimally.

Excess iron in the liver may hurt it. If there is too much iron, it may overwhelm the proteins designed to store it and then hurt other proteins which are not used to having so much of it around. Some clinical trials of interferon effectiveness have suggested that the patients with excess levels of iron in their livers do not respond as well to interferon as those with normal iron levels. Some physicians have committed their entire careers to this observation and trying to understand how best to help infected individuals in light of it.

It seems prudent that patients with hepatitis C become aware of their iron levels. If they have been bleeding and losing iron through their gastrointestinal tract, they may be anemic from iron deficiency. More likely, patients with chronic hepatitis C infection and often those who have already progressed to cirrhosis may have increased iron levels. Certainly someone who already has too much iron in their body does not need to take iron supplements; in fact such supplements could turn out to be harmful. Patients with markedly elevated iron levels may have the genetic disease hemochromatosis, which is an inherited defect in the ability to regulate iron absorption. For patients with very high iron levels, restricting the dietary intake of iron-rich foods such as bloody red meats and iron-enriched processed food products may be appropriate.

10

Hepatitis C and Interferon

Only when there is an easy and consistent cure for the hepatitis C virus, when every patient who is infected can be successfully treated, will problems caused by the virus become of less concern. Any person infected with hepatitis C should be optimistic about the possibilities for cures and treatments. When a cure will occur is difficult to say—for some people it is occurring right now; others may choose to wait for further advances or choose to enroll in experimental therapies. Certainly, no one with hepatitis C infection should ignore the infection or be lost to medical follow-up.

As we better understand how the immune system works, it is becoming easier to modulate the body's immune system to fight infection. Our immune system enables us to fight off many viral and bacterial infections without taking medicines. For some infections, like chronic hepatitis C, the immune system's attack is usually not sufficient to remove the infection from the body. The immune response is modulated by chemical messages which serve to stimulate or modulate the immune response to foreign invaders. Many of these chemical messages, or cytokines, have been identified and characterized and interferon is an example of these immune stimulatory chemical messengers that is useful as a drug.

Interferon is used as an anticancer as well as an antiviral agent. As important as its use is in the treatment of hepatitis, cancer treatment accounts for almost half of the applications of this remarkable immune modulator. The drug is approved for use in more than a dozen different diseases including treatment of chronic hepatitis B, chronic hepatitis C, hairy cell leukemia, AIDS-related Kaposi's sarcoma, and condylomata acuminata (venereal warts), and as adjuvant or booster therapy for malignant melanoma. For example, people with malignant melanoma are often treated with interferon as an adjuvant, or response-boosting, treatment prior to surgery. Malignant melanoma is a potentially fatal skin cancer. Surgical removal of the tumors is the only known cure, but surgical removal is not always effective if the tumors are too large or too deep. Interferon actually shrinks skin tumors by boosting the immune response against these lesions. The drug is used as an adjuvant to surgery, increasing the success of the surgery in a group of patients with melanoma. Interferon is also used in combination with chemotherapy to treat other forms of cancer. More traditional chemotherapies attack tumors directly. Interferon boosts the body's own immune system to attack the tumors. By using more than one drug that acts through different mechanisms, the cancer treatment may be more effective. When used in conjunction with other forms of chemotherapy, interferon has been shown to prolong survival in select groups of people with non-Hodgkin's lymphoma, a specific type of cancer. In a large randomized clinical study conducted at 31 medical centers between 1986 and 1991, patients with advanced-stage follicular lymphoma received either chemotherapy or chemotherapy plus interferon. Following a 6-year follow-up, the patients treated with chemotherapy plus interferon showed a significantly longer cancer progression-free survival (2.9 years versus 1.5 years) and a significantly longer overall survival (median not yet reached versus 5.6 years) than patients treated with chemotherapy alone. Similar approaches using interferon in combination with other anti–hepatitis C drugs are now fashionable.

Interferon is also used to treat people with chronic hepatitis B. Interferon was actually used to treat chronic hepatitis B–infected individuals even before hepatitis C was discovered. In people with low viral loads and active inflammation, the success rate for clearing active viral infection with hepatitis B approaches 40% in this select patient group having chronic active hepatitis B.

What is interferon, anyway? Interferon is a cytokine, which is a kind of naturally occurring protein which stimulates or augments an immune response to a foreign infection. Proteins are molecules that carry out all of the metabolic roles in the body. They are composed of amino acids, which are like the molecular building blocks of proteins. Hundreds of these amino acids are linked together in long chains to form protein molecules. Many classical drugs are not proteins but much smaller, man-made chemicals. In contrast, the cytokine interferon is a protein that occurs normally in our cells; scientists have figured out how to make it and deliver it to people with diseases.

Using proteins as drugs faces challenges. One challenge is delivering the protein to its active site. Another is having it remain intact while circulating in the blood. The blood contains many proteases, which are molecules designed to degrade circulating proteins. Therefore, the second that interferon is injected into the body, proteases begin breaking it down. This cleavage of interferon into its constituent building-block amino acids limits the duration of activity of the interferon molecule. If we could design an interferon substance more resistant to breakdown, the molecule might have an extended period of activity, thereby increasing its efficacy at stimulating the immune system to clear the hepatitis C virus.

Several methods are being attempted to extend interferon's life in the body. One method involves attaching the interferon to a molecule called polyethylene glycol, or PEG, to stabilize it. This is a time-tested technique which has been used to stabilize other proteins in the blood so that they do not break down so quickly, and has been shown to prolong interferon's durability in the bloodstream. Attaching interferon to PEG is like putting training wheels on a youngster's bike; the ride lasts longer and is more stable with the wheels in place. PEG may certainly pose some potential advantages in interferon administration, which makes it an exciting area of research. Other ideas include delivering interferon directly to the liver or to special immune cells, called antigen-presenting cells. These cells are professionals, dedicated to stimulating the immune response to foreign infections. If these cells could be infected with the hepatitis C virus and stimulated with interferon, the immune response might be more robust than occurs naturally. All these methods of extending the activity of interferon are very exciting, and interferon is the cornerstone of present-day therapy for hepatitis C. Naturally, developing new therapies takes time. The FDA requires careful tests of drug effectiveness before new concepts can be brought to market. These clinical trials are also expensive, requiring the cooperation of many patients and clinical investigators.

Interferon is currently used for the treatment of hepatitis C as an injection under the skin (subcutaneous injection). The injections are usually given in the thigh or abdomen. People need to be trained in the proper techniques of sterile injection. At times, redness and swelling may occur at the injection site. It is important to be alert for signs of infection. Some interferon manufacturers sell the drug in prefilled syringes to avoid the necessity of having to draw up the dose of medicine from a bottle.

Recently, a penlike interferon injector has been brought to the market (the Intron A Multidose Pen, manufactured by Schering-Plough). This device is preloaded with interferon, and the hepatitis C-infected individual dials up the prescribed dose of medicine. The device contains a reservoir of interferon in the barrel of the pen, a pop-up dosage scale, and a push

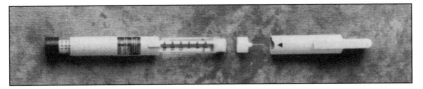

Figure 5. Intron A Multidose Pen. The multidose pen was developed to simplify interferon injections given to treat hepatitis C. It eliminates the need to draw up medicine from a vial into a syringe with a needle, measure it, and keep the separate medicine bottle sterile for repeated use. The simplified system allows the individual to dial in their prescribed dose, mitigating the chance of dosing errors. Since the pen contains medicine, it should be stored refrigerated between uses to keep the medicine fresh. (Picture: Schering-Plough)

button formed by the pop-up dosage scale once the desired dose has been selected. The needle attaches to the barrel of the pen. The pens are available in three concentrations of interferon; they are color-coded to avoid confusion. Injections can be given until the unit runs out of medicine, at which time it is discarded and replaced with a similar unit. In between uses, the multidose pen should be refrigerated to preserve the interferon.

The routine dose of interferon consists of 3 million units injected three times weekly. This dose was arrived at because it worked in an initial pilot study of interferon in treating non-A, non-B, transfusion-associated hepatitis performed by Dr. Jay Hoofnagle at the National Institutes of Health. It is remarkable that interferon treatment was discovered in 1986, even before the hepatitis C virus, the cause of most cases of non-A, non-B hepatitis. Follow-up studies have confirmed the essence of this seminal small pilot study, so Dr. Hoofnagle's observation that a significant fraction of treated hepatitis C-infected individuals may be cured with interferon treatment is well established. Follow-up studies have placed this interferon cure rate at 10–20% of hepatitis C-infected individuals.

One question that comes up is whether 3 million units three times a week is the optimal dose of interferon. Interferon is used to treat several other conditions, including cancer and chronic hepatitis B, at much higher doses (as great as 9 million units a day) than those used routinely for hepatitis C. Naturally, many of the side effects of interferon are dose dependent; the incidence of decreased white blood counts and flulike symptoms such as headache, muscle aches, fatigue, and fever goes up with increasing doses of interferon. It is not unusual for individuals using interferon to notice a decreased appetite, and treated individuals may lose 10 to 20 pounds over the 1-year treatment course without alarm.

Several studies are under way to determine whether a higher dose of interferon may increase the percent of individuals responding to treatment. One provocative concept is whether higher doses may be used in the beginning of a treatment program with the doses reduced later in the treatment period. These regimens are analogous to cancer treatment protocols in which there is an induction period followed by a consolidation period of treatment. The hope is that the toxicities of high-dose treatment may be tolerated for a brief period of time, permitting the benefits of high dose treatment and minimizing the side effects.

Initially, the drug was administered for 6 consecutive months as a standard length of treatment. Now, the routine treatment course is a full year. This longer treatment course

Table 8.   Side Effects of Interferon

Common	Rare
Joint and muscle aches	Seizures
Fevers	Suicide
Headache	Pronounced depression
Hair loss	Loose stools
Thyroid disease, autoimmune disease	
Nausea	
Lassitude	
Weight loss	
Irritability	

results in a higher percentage of people maintaining a sustained response to interferon once the drug has been stopped. This observation was arrived at by a number of clinical trials. When used to fight hepatitis C, individual responses to interferon treatment may be divided into three broad categories: (1) sustained responders, who rid the virus from their blood and have their serum liver enzymes return to normal even 6 months after therapy is stopped; (2) nonresponders, who do not show a disappearance of viral RNA levels from the blood and do not have their serum liver enzymes return to normal; and (3) partial responders, who drop their viral levels and liver enzymes on treatment but fail to maintain those successes once treatment is discontinued.

Since we have defined a sustained response as being free of the virus 6 months after infection, the critical question is whether these infected people are really cured long term and is the progression to cirrhosis aborted. Preliminary studies suggest that the answer is an emphatic *yes.* People who maintain a sustained response to interferon after 6 months off treatment do not get reinfected with the virus. They also do not progress further to cirrhosis. In a study of patients treated with interferon between 1984 and 1987, Dr. Hoofnagle and his colleagues discovered that all of the patients who had a sustained response remained HCV-free at an average of 10 years after therapy. Fibrosis had improved, and the HCV infection had not come back. The fact that fibrosis can improve when the infection is cured is particularly good news. In short, these people did not have liver disease 10 years after they had been cured of their hepatitis C infection.

People in the same study who were treated with interferon but did not achieve a sustained response had symptoms of chronic hepatitis on long-term follow-up and clearly fared worse than those cured of the virus. They generally had progression of fibrosis or scarring of the liver. Some progressed to end-stage liver disease.

One other question that comes to mind is whether treatment with interferon is beneficial even if it does not clear the viral infection. Many individuals exhibit a transient or partial response to interferon treatment, and one question being actively investigated in ongoing clinical trials is whether suppressing viral RNA levels and serum liver enzymes in the absence of a cure of the hepatitis C infection will be of long-term benefit to the patient. One of the problems in obtaining answers to these questions is that the end point in which we are interested may be decades away from the time of treatment. This is one reason why many of these clinical studies are extremely expensive and difficult to perform—patients must be maintained in follow-up for a long time. Because we want to find out as quickly as possible what may prolong hepatitis C-infected patients' lives, quite often surrogate markers such as the rate of increase in fibrosis in the liver or the rate of increase in symptoms may be used rather than simply assessing longevity on or off treatment. As these studies progress over years, we are learning more about the benefits and disadvantages to treatments that suppress but do not eliminate the virus.

Who is most likely to respond to interferon? Two of the best predictors of future response to interferon are the viral load (amount of virus in the serum) and the amount of fibrosis on the liver biopsy. People with chronic hepatitis C infection usually have high levels of circulating virus in their serum. For instance, the lower limit of detection of hepatitis C-RNA by the Chiron branched DNA signal amplification method is 0.20 mEq (1 mEq = 1×10^6 equivalents/mL). (A patient with 1 mEq has 1 million viral particles circulating per 1 milliliter of his serum). The more virus in the blood, the harder it is to get rid of it. The more advanced the scarring in the liver, the less likely interferon is to clear the infection. Women, people who have been infected for a shorter period of time, and younger people all have an improved chance at achieving a sustained response.

Who don't we treat with interferon? People who are actively drinking alcohol or abusing drugs. The response rate is less, and lack of compliance with the interferon regimen is a major problem; better to be clean and sober before starting treatment. Patients with decompensated cirrhosis are not treated either; they are much less likely to have a beneficial response and much more likely to run up against problems with treatment. Patients with a history of prior suicide attempts or major psychiatric disorders are not treated either; again the goal here is to do no harm. Patients with preexisting significant autoimmune disorders are also not treated with interferon as this may exacerbate their underlying disease. Finally, patients who have a low platelet count (platelets clot blood) or low white blood count (white blood cells fight infections) must be treated with great care if at all, as interferon can further decrease these important blood components. Many physicians defer treating patients who have no inflammatory activity on their liver biopsy or normal serum liver enzymes.

At present, interferon treatment is recommended for eligible patients with elevated serum liver enzymes, evidence of hepatitis C infection on serum antibody and/or RNA tests, and a liver biopsy consistent with hepatitis C infection (active inflammation characteristic of hepatitis C infection and fibrosis). One other important group of individuals is those who have normal serum liver enzymes. These individuals may well have significant liver damage on biopsy, but their serum liver enzyme tests are currently within the normal range. Long-term studies suggest these individuals may progress at a slower rate than those who have active elevations in their serum liver enzyme tests. As these patients with normal liver enzymes are followed, many of them tend to develop serum liver enzyme elevations over time. While the evidence compelling someone to treat individuals with normal liver enzymes is less strong than treating those with elevated liver enzymes, there is some rationale for treating these people as well. For example, younger people tend to respond better to interferon treatment, so why wait for progression? As better treatments are developed, patients with normal liver enzymes and hepatitis C infection may well be treated as aggressively as those who already have elevated enzymes. In the interim, the decision to treat hepatitis C-infected individuals with normal liver enzymes is made on a case-by-case basis.

DIFFERENT FORMS OF INTERFERON ARE AVAILABLE

One area which deserves special mention is the use of multiple forms of interferon. Interferon alpha 2b, Schering Plough's Intron A, was the first interferon approved for use in treating hepatitis C. Subsequently another manufacturer, Roche Pharmaceuticals, got approval to manufacture interferon alpha 2a for hepatitis C treatment. While these products are quite similar, there are subtle differences in their preparation. They are manufactured by two different companies, and there are a variety of papers supporting the use of one form or another of this compound. Yet another approach was to recognize that there are a variety of subtly different interferon molecules in the body, and to develop a consensus interferon with homology to all the different forms. This consensus interferon is marketed by Amgen; a variety of papers purport to demonstrate advantages to its use. In theory there should not be a major benefit of one form or another, and most clinical trials have not disclosed any such benefit. Several other companies are studying their own interferons, which are not currently approved by the FDA.

COMBINATION THERAPIES FOR HEPATITIS C

Great strides are being made in the use of combination therapies to treat hepatitis C infection, most strikingly with therapies combining interferon and ribavirin. Ribavirin is a medicine that is similar in structure to the building blocks for RNA, nucleosides. RNA is the genetic information used by the virus to store the information on how to make copies of itself; it is like the virus' computer program. Ribavirin has activity against hepatitis C; it is an antiviral compound, but the exact way it disrupts the virus is not well defined. While interferon is given in shots under the skin, ribavirin is an easier medicine to take as it comes in more traditional pills, which are swallowed. The usual current dosage of ribavirin is either 1000 mg/day for individuals less than 75 kg, or 1200 mg/day for those weighing 75 kg or more. Ribavirin pills are usually prescribed in split dosing, once in the morning and once in the evening. While interferon monotherapy has been shown to cure 10–20% of people with hepatitis C infection, the addition of ribavirin has increased the rate of elimination of the virus from previously infected people at the end of and 6 months after the study is over, up to approximately 30–40% in patients enrolled in protocols. These encouraging studies are being performed both in interferon-naïve people, i.e., those who have not been treated before, and in people who have not responded to interferon. The drug combination appears to benefit both groups. The use of interferon in combination with ribavirin is being applied more broadly to patients infected with hepatitis C who are not enrolled in experimental protocols now.

It is remarkable that ribavirin works, even though we do not know the mechanism of its action. We know that it is an antiviral compound which has worked against some other viruses, but its application to treat hepatitis C infection is strictly a result of empirical testing. We know that ribavirin alone does not have a sustained benefit to the hepatitis C patient. Nevertheless, the combination of interferon and ribavirin has proved quite beneficial.

One concern when using interferon or ribavirin or the combination of the two is medication side effects or toxicities. The side effects of interferon and ribavirin treatments are apparently additive. In other words, there is really no change in the side-effects profile of the combination other than the addition of the side effects of interferon to the side effects of ribavirin. Interferon's most common side effects include a lowered white blood count (which can make people more susceptible to infection), fatigue, muscle aches, headaches, fever, chills and, rarely, an increased serum liver enzyme, AST. Other frequently occurring side effects include nausea, vomiting, depression, hair loss, diarrhea, and lowered platelet counts. The most concerning, and thankfully very infrequent, side effect reported with interferon is suicidal tendencies, including suicidal thoughts, suicide attempts, and, more rarely, suicide. Interferon has also been shown to modestly increase the susceptibility to seizures; this may be of concern in people with a preexisting seizure disorder. Still other side effects include flulike symptoms of fever, muscle aches, and somnolence. There can also be problems with discomfort at the site of injection, and headaches.

Among the most serious potential side effects, the lowering of the white blood count renders the individual much more susceptible to other infections, or the platelet count may drop, leading to bleeding tendencies. Finally, the drug may even cause worsening of decompensated, end-stage liver disease in the setting of hepatitis C infection. As mentioned, the drug also lowers the seizure threshold and can sometimes, albeit rarely, precipitate grand mal seizures in susceptible individuals, such as those who already have epilepsy.

Ribavirin has two primary side effects of concern. The first and most common is hemolysis. Ribavirin is concentrated inside red blood cells in the body. As it affects these red blood cells, they are prone to break or rupture. This weakening of red cells leading to their breakdown, hemolysis, can make people undergoing treatment with ribavirin anemic. This anemia, or lowered hematocrit, leads to a decreased oxygen-carrying capacity in the blood. Blood counts can fall as much as 20% on ribavirin treatment, which is particularly dangerous in people with preexisting cardiovascular or cerebrovascular disease. Since ribavirin is cleared from the body through the kidneys, people with kidney problems need to be particularly careful with this drug. Rapid falls in blood counts can be associated with myocardial infarction or heart attack, as well as potential for stroke. Because of these concerns, some advocate pretreatment cardiac stress testing for those who receive ribavirin therapy. Nevertheless, there have only been a few reports of heart attacks in people taking ribavirin in FDA-sanctioned preapproval trials. As the drug is now being prescribed by physicians outside the guise of clinical trials, care will have to be used in patients predisposed to heart disease. Any strokes or heart attacks that occur during treatment will need to be followed carefully to be sure they are not happening at a greater-than-anticipated rate.

The second most common side effect of ribavirin is also cause for concern. Ribavirin has been shown to be a teratogen, meaning that *it can cause birth defects in the offspring of men and women taking the drug.* In animal studies, observed drug-induced malformations included changes in the skull, jaw, palate, eye, limbs, skeleton, and gastrointestinal tract. These deformities occurred at doses of the medicine lower than those used in human therapy. Giving the drug to people of childbearing age necessitates the judicious use of prophylactic contraception during the time of ribavirin use by a treated male or a treated female. When engaging in intercourse, both partners need to use a contraceptive device. Even with the careful use of contraceptives, people may conceive secondary to condom rupture or diaphragm failure, etc., which may lead to the birth of offspring with ribavirin-induced deformities.

At the present time, the side effects of these two medications appear to be additive not synergistic, and therefore no new side effects have been discovered which are not seen with either one drug or the other. This is certainly cause for optimism, as it is always a concern that drug interactions may lead to more serious side effects.

"Rebetron" is the trademark name for combination therapy with ribavirin and interferon. Rebetron is marketed by Schering-Plough, and these medications come in combination packages containing the ribavirin capsules and interferon a-2b, so that the only way to purchase them is together. The dosage used involves 3 million units three times weekly of interferon A, and 1000–1200 mg/day in divided doses of ribavirin, based on an individual's weight.

It is important to note that male individuals taking this combined regimen should practice contraception during and for 6 months after treatment. Similarly, women of childbearing potential need to use safe contraception during the treatment period and for 6 months posttherapy. This recommendation is based on the long duration or half-life of ribavirin in the blood. It turns out that ribavirin is concentrated inside red blood cells and may circulate in the serum, decreasing levels by half only every 12 days. The concern about use of these drugs in the setting of pregnancy or potential pregnancy is that ribavirin produces dramatic teratogenic effects (congenital deformations) in all animal species in which studies have been conducted, including malformations of the skull, palate, eye, jaw, limbs, skeleton, and GI tract. The incidence and severity of teratogenic effects are dose dependent. In its most severe forms, this teratogenesis can cause the death of the fetus or offspring. As noted before, men are advised to use contraception during ribavirin treatment because ribavirin can be contained in sperm; whether it could have a teratogenic effect on ova at fertilization is unknown.

Other potential toxicities of interferon treatment include accumulation in people who have poor renal function, the induction of diabetes or hyperglycemia in people treated with interferon and in rare cases retinal hemorrhages. In addition, there have been reports of hypersensitivity or allergic reactions including severe reactions where the blood pressure falls (anaphylaxis), constriction of the airways in the lungs, swelling of the limbs, and an allergic, itching rash. Finally, interferon has been shown to induce autoimmune thyroid abnormalities during treatment, and thus thyroid function needs to be monitored so that if hyperthyroidism develops it may be treated medically.

The first FDA-approved treatment course for combination therapy was for hepatitis C-infected people who have not responded to interferon monotherapy as the initial line of treatment. Next, Schering-Plough received broader FDA approval for an additional treatment indication; they have achieved accelerated approval for treatment with combination interferon and ribavirin therapy for individuals who have never taken interferon before. While the data are much more dramatic from treating people who have not responded to interferon alone with combination therapy, the data also appear to support an improved benefit in maintaining people in sustained response when treated with a combination of interferon with ribavirin as opposed to interferon alone. The Food and Drug Administration weighed the evidence of improved response rates along with the increased toxicities in making its decision to approve combination therapy for interferon-naïve individuals.

Rebertron is not cheap. At one pharmacy, the cost of a 6-month course of therapy is approximately $9000. Why does it cost so much? In short, the clinical trials necessary to bring Rebertron to market can cost about $30 million per study. There also are tremendous marketing costs involved in the launch of a new product. Physicians, pharmacists, and individuals infected with the virus need to be educated by product detailers. For all new drugs, pharmaceutical companies need to generate strong outcome data to prove that their product is worth prescribing and that insurance companies or health maintenance organizations should pay for it. There are liability issues involved with marketing any combination drug with a significant side-effects profile. Finally, for every successful drug launched there are scores of failures, drugs which initially look promising but do not pan out. The cost of developing these market losers must be absorbed in the cost of the medicine. Dr. Bates knew, but $9000? He was staggered. As it turns out, the time of patent protection for ribavirin in combination with interferon is relatively short, so the company must recoup its costs in a relatively short period of time before the patent protection expires and generic alternatives become available. Fortunately, many patients have insurance policies that cover the costs of treatment and the company has indigent care programs.

The kinetics or time course of interferon/ribavirin action appear to be different from the kinetics of interferon monotherapy. Some have advocated an initial 12-week treatment period for interferon monotherapy to sort out responders from nonresponders, discontinuing treatment in nonresponders to spare costs and toxicities. With combination therapy, on the other hand, it appears that a significant number of people may respond after 12 weeks who failed to respond initially. This lag in response may relate to the time necessary to accumulate therapeutic levels of ribavirin in the body. The optimal duration of treatment for the combination regimen has also not been determined just yet. The drug was initially approved for 6 months of therapy only, but data with interferon monotherapy suggest that a year of treatment may prove better at holding a higher percentage of people in complete response. Further studies are under way to address this issue of duration of treatment, and some suggest a benefit to treating with combination therapy for one year.

It should be noted that the risk of hemolysis appears to be greater in people over 50 years old. Why would this be? Perhaps it relates to the decrease in kidney function with age. Since ribavirin is eliminated by the kidneys, it may accumulate in the body more readily in older people, who tend to have a lower renal clearance. As the drug builds up, hemolysis increases as the risk of hemolysis appears to be dose related. The dose of ribavarin can be adjusted or reduced depending on the side effects.

Another hopeful area of research involves what is termed induction therapy with interferon. This is where much higher doses are given in order to achieve a response to the medication. This may be as high as 5 million or 7 million units per day. This is an area of ongoing investigation; obviously the side effects of interferon are greater at the higher dose. One note of caution is that interferon must always be monitored carefully through blood tests to assess liver functions as well as white blood cell and platelet counts. The most common mistake made by people taking interferon is to not take this blood testing seriously. Bleeding, dangerous infections or, rarely, particularly in people with preexisting cirrhosis, worsening liver disease can be missed if patients don't get monitored.

Another concern in the treatment of hepatitis C virus is the development of resistant strains of the virus to interferon or other antivirals. One benefit of using combination therapy is that it may be possible to eradicate the virus more quickly before resistant strains develop. Potential comparisons to be made are with resistant strains of HIV, bacterial infections or even tuberculosis that are developed while taking anti-infective therapy. For this reason future therapies will probably use additional combinations of drugs that are under development. One reason the development of resistant strains is a concern is that multiple mutations occur in the virus as time progresses. The set of instructions the virus uses to reproduce itself and make its proteins (viral genome) is highly mutable, and the virus is constantly changing its proteins to evade immune attack. These kinds of changes also occur against antiviral compounds, which can be problematic as well. The ideal antiviral compound would work against a drug target, which is essential in its native, or unchanged, form for viral survival. In this way any mutations that occur that could confer antiviral resistance would lead to death of the virus.

One drug target that has received intense scrutiny is the viral protease, which functions to separate some of the viral proteins to allow for proper virus function. This protease is therefore essential for hepatitis C replication and survival. Analogies can be drawn with HIV; development of antiviral compounds to the HIV protease led to a marked benefit in the treatment of this tragic viral infection. It is hoped that protease inhibitors for hepatitis C will have a similar dramatic impact on this disease.

The use of antiviral compounds in the treatment of hepatitis C virus will no doubt increase. The best current regimens cure 30–40% of people selected for clinical protocols, which still leaves a large percentage of hepatitis C-infected individuals who do not respond to therapy in need of a cure. Research is ongoing into compounds that attack the hepatitis C virus directly, compounds that boost the body's own immune system to attack the virus and compounds that will attack some of the pathophysiology of the disease. One example of attacking the liver injury caused by infection involves developing compounds which prevent either fibrosis (scarring over of the liver), or actual fibrinolytics, which break down the fibrotic tissue once it has formed. Naturally, cirrhosis is one of the most troubling side effects of hepatitis C infection, and if compounds could be developed that either prevented or reversed cirrhosis, this would be a major breakthrough in the symptomatic treatment of hepatitis C infection.

In summary, certainly, treating chronic hepatitis C is a challenge. Though doctors have had some modest successes, the future seems more promising. Future improvements include optimized dosing schedules to deliver the best amount of the drugs we already know have some benefits for the correct amount of time. Improved immune regulatory molecules or delivery systems, such as binding interferon to PEG or testing other molecules similar in action but potentially synergistic in activity to interferon, hold promise. Finally, new classes of drugs, like hepatitis C viral protease inhibitors, are being studied attentively. Other antiviral drugs, like ribavirin, also contribute to the armamentarium against hepatitis C in the form of combination therapy with interferon. Only through careful laboratory research in combination with judicious clinical trials will these advances be brought to fruition.

11

Alternative Medicine or Unconventional Medicine

Since conventional treatments for hepatitis fail for many, a number of infected people have felt motivated to explore treatments outside the realm of traditional Western medicine. These may include herbs, spices, extreme diets, vitamins, chemical antioxidants, and medicines not approved for use in this country. Over 3% of the United States population has tried herbal remedies at one time or another.

There is a growing effort to accept certain herbal and home treatments as useful. For many, this will require evidence-based research which demonstrates an improved outcome, such as clearance of hepatitis C infection, while using a particular home remedy. Not long ago, these treatments were quickly dismissed as quackery by many physicians in this country. The specialist in Western medicine might have pictured a sick, vulnerable individual being preyed on by a slick herbalist in a monklike robe. While physicians like Dr. Bates have become a little more open-minded about herbal treatments, there remains a vast chasm between Eastern and Western medical practices and teachings.

While these types of treatment have been popularly labeled alternative medicine, the label unconventional medicine is in many ways more accurate for many of these treatments. The word alternative implies that there is at least some body of data to suggest that a given treatment may be beneficial or is indeed a sound medical practice. Another moniker attached to these treatments is to call them "complementary," implying in some way that there is a positive interaction between Eastern and Western medical practices. This name is particularly dangerous as interactions between herbs and interferon have not been well studied; such mixtures are strictly experimental. The potential for additive or synergistic side effects exists.

Many of these treatments can best be labeled unconventional as they are practiced with scant or no scientific or outcomes-oriented research to support their use. Suffice it to say there are no miracle cures here, but it would be equally inaccurate to categorize all of unconventional medicine in a class with a post–Civil War era carpet bagger's "snake oil," which was billed to cure whatever ails you. Many of these treatments have at least a modicum of rationale behind their use. There is a growing trend to try to develop outcomes-based research using unconventional treatments, and the federal government is funding research into potentially beneficial unconventional remedies through the National Institutes of Health.

The alternative or unconventional treatments people seek have included many herbal and other home remedies. One of the most fashionable is milk thistle. This is an extract of the milk thistle plant and is taken orally. Some patients on milk thistle have actually been noted to have lowered serum liver chemistries, which is somewhat encouraging, but there have been no scientific studies to prove its effectiveness at combating hepatitis C or to clearly define its hazards.

Dr. Bates was not aware of anyone who has cured their hepatitis C infection using any of these unconventional treatments. In some confidential patient questionings, over half the patients with hepatitis C are noted to have experimented with home remedies at some time during their illness. For this reason Dr. Bates often asks people what home remedies they are using and what herbs they are taking rather than asking them whether they are using any. People are often reluctant to discuss their home remedies with medical practitioners, which is unfortunate. Herbs are really used by everyone, since we all eat vegetables and certain spices. As a vegetarian, Dr. Bates appreciated many of the benefits that herbs can confer.

Nevertheless, herbs can also be dangerous. This danger can come from many different sources. First of all, the drugs we buy through the pharmacy have all gone through clinical trials and been approved by the Food and Drug Administration. They have passed studies in Phase I, Phase II, and Phase III clinical trials which document the toxicity, side effects, effectiveness and drug interactions of these medications. Physicians and patients therefore have a ready reference to study when seeking out rare or unusual drug side effects. With herbs, on the other hand, such data are far more elusive. Herbs consist of a mixture of many different compounds. The heterogeneous spectrum of chemicals in herbs and plants and plant variability make it harder to study side effects and interactions than with traditional, FDA-approved pharmaceuticals. This is because mixtures of compounds which vary from one bottle to the next with multiple "active" ingredients can generate less consistent side effects than pure drugs. Furthermore, pharmaceutical compounds are studied in tremendous detail to assay their purity, consistency, and quality from one batch or production run to another. Herbs, because they grow wild, under uncontrolled conditions, show a tremendous amount of batch-to-batch variability. Many herbs are available by mail order or over the Internet with little or no control on their source, authenticity, purity, or possible side effects. Some companies have responded to this concern by placing "purity" seals on their herbs. Let the buyer beware—variability is part of the organic nature of plants and herbs.

Certainly people consuming herbs expose themselves to the risks from batch-to-batch variability. Plants grown in one section of China, for example, may have different characteristics and varying effects from plants of the same species grown in another section of China. Seasonal changes in light and rain affect the harvest of any crop. Oftentimes people go to tremendous lengths to obtain appropriate metal-free herbal pots in which to brew their herbs at home, and may pursue an almost ritualistic practice of brewing seven or eight different teas throughout the course of the day to treat their own liver disease.

The most important caveat to follow is to recognize the dangers of a contaminated or inconsistent herbal supply and to recognize the need for discontinuing these herbs at times if liver disease worsens in order to evaluate their effects on the liver. There needs to be good communication between patient and physician with regard to the herbs that are being used.

The overall safety record of Chinese herbal remedies is strikingly good. Serious poisoning can occur in some susceptible individuals, and certain preparations have been associated with liver injury (see Table 9, above). *Jin Bu Huan Anodyne* tablets are a Chinese herbal medicine used to relieve pain. They have been used in the United States for more than a decade with 7 cases of acute herb-induced liver inflammation diagnosed. Several individuals who could not believe that the herb could be the cause took the herb again and got sick again. None of the cases involved an overdose of the herb; all were taking the amount prescribed by an herbalist. Sho-saiko-to is particularly alarming because it is used for chronic hepatitis in Japanese herbal therapy even though it can cause hepatitis. Possible toxicities include fibrosis or scarring of the liver, liver cell death and fatty accumulation in the liver. Individuals should think twice before taking these herbs with known liver toxicity, particularly while attempting treatment for hepatitis C. If liver injury occurs, it may prove difficult to figure out if the

Table 9. Herbal Remedies to Avoid in Hepatitis C Infection

Remedy	Prescribed for	Liver damage
Sho-saiko-to (traditional Japanese)	Chronic viral hepatitis	Liver death, fibrosis
Jin Bu Huan Anodyne (Chinese herbal)	Sedative, pain killer	Hepatitis, fibrosis
Glycyrrhizin (Chinese herbal)	Chronic hepatitis	Vanishing bile duct syndrome[a]
Oil of cloves	Pain	Liver death
Comfrey tea	Health tonic	Veno-occlusive disease[b]
T'usanchi'i (Chinese herbal)	Health tonic	Veno-occlusive disease[b]

[a]Disappearance of bile ducts from liver.
[b]Clotting off of blood vessels in liver.

hepatitis C is progressing, or whether a herb had a deleterious side effect. Clearly these herbs can prove to be dangerous.

It is important both that the hepatitis C-infected individual not be overzealous and believe automatically that herbs can do no harm, and that the physician not give a knee jerk response and believe that herbs can never do any good. Obviously if herbal remedies routinely cured this disease, this would be widely known. Anecdotal Internet success stories should be viewed with skepticism. For this reason Dr. Bates does not recommend that people take herbs for treatment but, should they choose to, it is important that they communicate their regimen to their physician. After all, the physician needs to take this into account when prescribing pharmaceutical drugs. Dr. Bates recognizes that many people infected with hepatitis C experiment on themselves with herbs. If patients feel strongly compelled to use herbs, Dr. Bates suggests milk thistle, but always with the warning that he knows of one case of liver death in an individual on milk thistle. It is also important that infected people understand that "natural" or herbal medicines are not automatically safe medicines. After all, many poisons are "natural."

12

The Body's Efforts to Fight Hepatitis C, and Potential Vaccines

So what do we think is happening when the virus infects someone? Initially, the virus circulates in the blood until it reaches the liver. Exactly how it gets inside liver cells is a matter of speculation. Some think the virus is coated with serum proteins, with its outer-coat, or envelope, proteins binding to the outside of liver cells as a first step in gaining entry to these cells. The exact way hepatitis C gets into cells has not been completely figured out; once it is known, drugs may be developed to block the virus from getting into cells. Once bound to the cell surface, the virus is taken up inside of the cell, perhaps by being surrounded first by snippets of the cell membrane, or outer boundary, of the cell. The virus makes copies of itself inside of liver cells. At least some of the infected

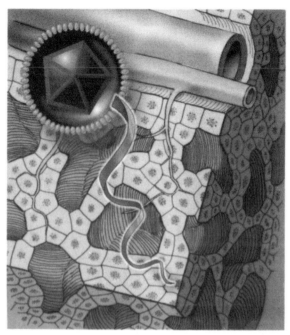

Figure 6.   The hepatitis C virus infecting liver cells. The virus particle has an envelope or coat with the virus RNA or instructions for making viral proteins fitting inside the envelope much as a letter fits inside a regular envelope (upper left). As the liver is infected, the RNA from the virus enters the cells (spiral structure connecting viral particle to the cells). Once inside, the virus replicates or copies itself using the instructions in the form of viral RNA to make numerous other virus particles, which are capable of infecting additional liver cells. Eventually, the virus infection spreads throughout the liver, causing damage to the liver cells over a long period of time, often several decades.

liver cells are attacked by the immune system and die, releasing large numbers of virus particles which can infect even more liver cells. Surprisingly, large numbers of virus particles circulate in the bloodstream. The large numbers of viral particles that can be found in the blood are stunning, exceeding millions of hepatitis C viruses in a tiny drop of serum.

What does the body do to respond to this foreign intrusion? Surely the virus is not greeted with warm hospitality like a welcome house guest. There are a broad range of immune responses to the virus. The simplest to conceive is the formation of antibodies against the virus. Antibodies are molecules made by our immune system which bind to specific foreign invaders through distinct molecular interactions. This occurs when the foreign viral proteins are engulfed by special cells which chop the foreign invader up into little pieces and "show" these to the rest of the body's immune system through simple molecular pathways. These bound fragments of invading virus are chaperoned to the cell surface, where the body recognizes them as foreign enemies and mounts an immune response. This response can include the formation of antibodies, which stick to the invading viruses. These sticky antibodies can cripple or partially cripple the virus' ability to infect other cells. Since much has been said of the ability of hepatitis C to constantly change its outer-coat or envelope proteins and therefore evade the crippling effects of the immune response to infection, it is easy to underestimate the role of these antibodies in ridding the body of an acute infection of hepatitis C. The changing envelope proteins are like a fugitive on the 10-most-wanted list who changes his costume constantly to avoid recognition and capture. It certainly is reassuring that up to 15% of people infected with hepatitis C are able to clear the infection early on in the infection. In other patients, the antibodies formed to the coat or envelope proteins of hepatitis C may slow down the pace of the invading virus even as they fail to get rid of the foreign intruder.

What happens when hepatitis C manages to slip by the molecular antibody defenders? Does the immune system have an ability to see inside cells to tell if they are infected? Certainly. The body has developed a system whereby chopped-up pieces of virus made inside of cells are presented to the immune system along another avenue or molecular pathway similar to, but distinct from, the roadway used to make antibodies. As this pathway functions, molecular chaperones bind pieces of the chopped-up virus and escort them to the cell surface. This technique allows the immune system to see inside of cells and tell which ones are harboring the foreign invading virus. When the immune cells detect the foreign invaders, this favors development of special immune cells which attack the foreign invaders, adding another type of cellular weapon to the antibodies already discussed to attack the virus. These immune cells which attack the invading virus include the cytotoxic cells, which are immune cells capable of punching holes in and killing cells that are hiding infectious foreign viruses.

Why are these cells that attack the infection important? They are what enable us to clear viral infections from our bodies even if these infections have set up shop inside our cells. By allowing the immune system to see inside of cells, cellular warriors of the immune system allow us to get rid of viral infections even if they have slipped past antibody defenders. They can be viewed like the defensive secondary, stopping the opposing team even if it breaks through the lineman at the line of scrimmage.

Much of the pathology observed with hepatitis C may be related to this immune attack on infected cells. Fibrosis, or scarring of the liver, appears to be in part a consequence of the immune response to the hepatitis C-infected liver cells. Not surprisingly, much as interferon, a natural molecule, is used to treat the viral infection, the body changes its own molecules in response to the hepatitis C invasion. Since these interferonlike molecules, called cytokines, modulate the immune system, this shift in the body's own immune response is another effort of the body to boost its protective attack to hepatitis C infection.

Vaccines are one of the single greatest advances in medical technology in the last century. With the advent of many effective vaccines for numerous human plagues, we have almost developed an expectation that vaccines serve as an arsenal against infectious diseases. Nevertheless many of the diseases which were first attacked through vaccination—for example, smallpox, measles and polio—actually have characteristics that make them highly susceptible to vaccination. The tremendous success of vaccination to eradicate smallpox, in particular, is a result of not only a highly effective vaccine, but also the ability of humans to mount an effective clearing immune response to that virus and the lack of a human reservoir of infected, chronic carriers of that virus to transmit smallpox further. In other words, the stunning eradication of smallpox through vaccination is, unquestionably, one of the miracles of modern medicine. Nevertheless, it is easy to point out that such success may not be possible for every virus.

When HIV was first discovered, for instance, people felt that a vaccine would be easily developed. Difficulties in developing an AIDS vaccine have centered around the rapid mutation of the envelope proteins, which coat the outside of the virus. These proteins generally bind to cell surface receptors, which are like doors that allow viral entry into cells. By blocking entry of a virus into a cell, a vaccine that makes an antibody against the coat proteins may prove effective in preventing viral transmission. This is like locking a door to prevent a burglar from getting into your house.

The hepatitis B vaccine is one good example of a vaccine which functions to block viral entry into cells. This vaccine consists of a piece of the virus coat, a recombinant hepatitis B surface antigen, which is used to open the door into the cell. When injected into humans along with an adjuvant or compound that stimulates the immune system to take note of its presence, the hepatitis B surface protein vaccine generates a potent antibody response. The antibody binds to the hepatitis B surface antigen, which acts like a shroud preventing the virus from getting into the cell by blocking entrance through a molecular door. Most importantly, this antibody response protects an individual from catching hepatitis B virus infection. The presence of antibodies that bind to the hepatitis B surface antigen is sufficient to prevent transmission of the virus.

In contrast, hepatitis C is not an easy virus for which to make a vaccine. The surface proteins (envelope, or coat, proteins) are constantly mutating or changing, which leads to alterations in the viral surface proteins, not only from one person to the next, but also within any given individual. Therefore, antibodies that are generated to the viral envelope may not be protective against viral infection. Secondly, since the body is generally not able to clear itself of hepatitis C infection when it originally occurs, this leads to difficulties generating an immune response with a vaccine that will be effective. In other words, we are asking a vaccine to do something better than what occurs naturally, rather than mimicking an immune response which already occurs in nature. It is not possible merely to mimic the body's natural response to hepatitis C with a vaccine. It is necessary to actually generate a more effective or better immune response to the virus than would normally occur with a natural infection. For these reasons, the development of a hepatitis C vaccine has proved problematic. It is like the FBI trying to hunt a fugitive who is a master of disguises. When they circulate his picture, he just changes his appearance and then no one recognizes him.

A simple recombinant envelope vaccine for hepatitis C has been tried on chimpanzees. Unfortunately, this vaccine would protect only against 5 to 10 chimp infectious units of virus. In contrast, a unit of infected blood might contain many million infectious particles. In addition, this vaccine would also have difficulty protecting against the many different strains, or genotypes, of hepatitis C.

There is cause for optimism nonetheless. Recent advances in vaccine technology are leading to the development of a new class of vaccines. These are called *DNA* or *expressed vaccine* constructs. The idea here is a simple one: Rather than injecting a protein into the body to generate an immune response, a gene therapy approach is used, meaning a DNA molecule which carries instructions for making proteins is injected to generate an immune response. The cell is used to make the protein vaccine. This is done by injecting the cells with DNA instructions that explain to the cell how to make the vaccine. It is like giving the cell a computer program detailing how to make a protein vaccine. The big difference, then, is that the protein part of the vaccine is made inside of the cell, rather than the outside. When the protein is made or expressed inside

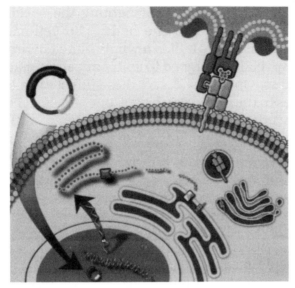

Figure 7. DNA vaccine. One exciting area of vaccine research involves using a gene therapy system to express snippets of hepatitis C inside of cells. The DNA vaccine is shown as a round circle of DNA (top left) which enters a cell (arrow) to generate or build a piece of virus inside the cell. The DNA makes RNA, which then is used to make proteins. These small snippets of noninfectious virus are then transported to the surface of the cell, where they interact with the immune system (upper right). This allows the immune system to better see the viral vaccine protein, thereby potentially mounting a more robust attack on an incipient or existing infection. The DNA vaccine in effect tricks the immune system to mount an attack on the piece of virus as if the body were being invaded by a foreign virus, when in actuality the DNA vaccine is safe and noninfectious. DNA vaccines fall into the category of experimental research.

the body, it is more efficiently presented to the immune system to generate a cell-mediated immune response.

Immune responses to foreign invaders can be split into two broad types: an antibody defense, which binds to the virus, and a cell-mediated defense, which consists of immune cells which attack the foreign invaders directly. Antibodies are like missiles fired out of cells that bind specifically to the foreign invaders. When the body is infected, it builds more missiles (antibodies) which are good at fighting the specific disease invader which challenges the body. The cell-mediated response is as if the body builds a whole bunch of armored cars which are specially designed to sniff out cells already infected with the virus. Once they detect these infected cells, they can punch holes in the cell's membrane, or outer surface, and fight the virus invaders. Vaccines can be engineered to stimulate the body to build an immune response which favors an antibody immune response or a cell-mediated response or both.

When a protein vaccine is injected into a person, it favors the development of an antibody immune response. The way viral molecules are processed by the immune system is different for proteins inside of cells from that for proteins outside of cells. This approach has been used to study DNA vaccines for influenza and for such dreaded viruses as the Ebola virus. It is hoped that use of these kinds of vaccines will provide technologies to battle diseases for which effective vaccines are not currently available.

The extent to which DNA vaccines will contribute to medical care remains to be determined. DNA vaccines work by delivering inside a cell the instructions or recipes (in the language of DNA) for a piece of the virus invader. The cell then reads these DNA instructions and *expresses*, or builds, this safe piece of the virus invader. While the virus piece by itself does not cause disease, the goal is that the immune response to the virus piece will direct the body to make antivirus missiles (antibodies) and antivirus-armored cars (cell-mediated immune response). These weapons then can either prevent a future infection by attacking the invader before it establishes a beachhead, or help bolster the attack on an existing infection. These DNA vaccines are the source of tremendous hope at this time, and there is a lot of ongoing study toward developing DNA vaccines for hepatitis C.

There is also a focus on new vaccine techniques, such as use of new adjuvants. Adjuvants are molecules which are injected along with the viral proteins to stimulate the body to generate an immune response. The traditional adjuvant used in animal immunization has been Freund's adjuvant. This agent, which boosts the immune response, is a cocktail of different particles, some of which are actually derived from the agent that causes tuberculosis. The cocktail is very potent in alerting the body to the fact that something foreign has invaded the area and that it needs to mount an immune response to it. Freund's adjuvant, unfortunately, causes too painful a swelling for use in human immunization. The main adjuvant used in immunization today is alum or an aluminum-containing compound. There is nonetheless a vigorous effort to establish alternative adjuvants, such as novel new lipid compounds which shuttle vaccines into cells almost as if they were made there. They may prove useful in generating an immune response.

One further area of emerging vaccine use which is very exciting is the use of vaccines as therapies. Vaccines have traditionally been thought of as prophylactic, or preventive, agents. In this use, vaccines are given to people that are healthy and they mount an immune response to the vaccine at the time of immunization. Because the body's immune system has a memory, at the time of infection with the wild-type virus, the individual then develops a more robust immune response to the infection than would have been possible had the person not been previously vaccinated.

The use of vaccines as therapies is now becoming more realistic. The concept here is to treat someone who already has the disease with a vaccine to boost the body's own immune system to that disease and permit the body to fight off the infection. In this way then, the vaccine works to augment the body's natural immune system to assist it in fighting infection, rather than developing a completely parallel treatment modality. The concept of boosting the body's own immune system to improve on a natural process of disease elimination is, obviously, quite enticing. It is encouraging, almost miraculous, that the use of interferon, a molecule that stimulates the body's own immune system, is able to cure even a small percentage of people infected with hepatitis C. Certainly anyone who has suffered with hepatitis C feels an uplifting sense of relief, almost joy, when they are told that the hepatitis C virus is no longer detectable in their body. In contrast, even the antiviral agents that are regarded as such an outstanding advance in the treatment of HIV, nucleoside analogs like AZT, never actually cure people of this disease at this time. Most important, interferon, on the other hand, which stimulates the body's immune system, can actually effect a cure. Therefore, there is growing optimism that if more effective ways can be established to boost the immune system of a previously infected individual, greater numbers of people may be cured of the hepatitis C viral infection.

How could therapeutic vaccination work? In this example, a person already infected with hepatitis C but whose immune response is not able to clear the viral infection would be vaccinated. After exposure to the vaccine, the body's own immune system would be further stimulated to fight off the hepatitis C infection, thereby allowing the person to be cured of infection. This may sound overly optimistic, but I think this optimism is justified. Certainly the fact that interferon is able to cure at least a small percentage of people with this infection is a cause for optimism that a hepatitis C vaccine might also help.

13

Your Skin and Joints:
Effects of Hepatitis C Outside the Liver

Patients with liver disease may also develop a variety of skin lesions including bruises, reddened palms, and half-inch-size red spots which vaguely resemble the body of a small spider with legs projecting out at all sides. The ecchymoses or bruises can result from a variety of sources, including increased blood vessel fragility in chronic liver disease, decreased platelet counts, which are the first building blocks of blood clots, and decreased blood clotting factors, which are like the mortar that holds platelets together. We do not know why palms turn red (palmar erythema) in some people with advanced liver disease. Sometimes the palms turn red or people develop red skin spots or spiders even when there is no liver disease present, so these are not always findings specific for advanced liver disease (cirrhosis).

The red spots on skin which vaguely resemble spiders, spider angiomata, are the result of a confluence of small arteries and veins in the skin. When you press on these spots, they turn white only to turn red once again when blood flows into them. The development of these "spiders" involves the proliferation of blood vessels, evidently in response to messages in the blood which are also stimulating the few remaining liver cells to proliferate in response to liver dysfunction or failure. Rarely, these "spiders" can break, surprising the unsuspecting individual with more than anticipated bleeding. Should bleeding occur, it is usually easily controlled with prolonged pressure, although occasionally an emergency room visit is necessary to cauterize the bleeding vessels.

Another skin lesion that develops in the setting of chronic hepatitis C infection consists of an increased sensitivity to sun exposure, darkened facial skin pigmentation, increased fragility or decreased toughness of the skin, and occasionally tiny vesicles on the backs of the hands. These skin lesions, known as porphyria cutanea tardia, or PCT, are directly related to changes in which the body metabolizes porphyrins, breakdown products of heme. Heme is one of the oxygen-carrying components of blood, a breakdown product of hemoglobin which comes into play when old blood cells are used up and destroyed. Unfortunately, the lesions may be quite dramatic. This skin disorder is associated with excessive levels of iron in the liver. PCT may be seen with other liver diseases besides hepatitis C, and more rarely there is an inherited form of the disease as well. Recall the old medical practice of using leeches to remove blood from the sick, such as the famous picture of George Washington being treated by his physician. PCT is one of the few diseases still treated with blood-letting or phlebotomy to decrease the body stores of iron. People infected with hepatitis C who develop PCT should undergo phlebotomy to normalize their serum iron levels before embarking on a treatment course with interferon or combination therapy with interferon and another antiviral agent. In people who respond to interferon, however, treatment with antihepatitis C therapy can lead to the disappearance of these lesions.

Hepatitis C virus is infamous for being a liver disease, but the infection is also recognized to have a broad variety of effects throughout the body. While hepatitis C can indirectly affect a variety of vital body systems through liver dysfunction, some of the effects of hepatitis C outside the liver are actually a result of more direct effects of the virus.

For example, samples of fluid from inflamed joints have been shown to contain hepatitis C. Some of this inflammation may come from the deposition in the joint space of small pieces of hepatitis C virus along with antibodies made by the immune system against the virus. People infected with hepatitis C occasionally complain that they feel soreness in joints all over their body. The symptoms may fluctuate or be quite persistent. This is termed polyarticular arthritis because it affects more than one joint at a time. More than one joint is inflamed because the virus circulates in the blood, accessing all the joints. Often these symptoms can be controlled with anti-inflammatory medicines. Depending on how advanced the liver disease is, there may be a tendency to avoid nonsteroidal anti-inflammatory drugs if the person already has cirrhosis of the liver. Then alternative treatments for arthritis may be sought. Compounds that may be used include narcotic analgesics and other antiarthritic regimens. Often there is a general reluctance to use these compounds in people with hepatitis C, as there may be associated liver toxicities with them. Therefore decisions about how to treat hepatitis C-associated arthritis must be made by the doctor with each individual depending on the severity of symptoms, severity of liver disease and associated pathology in the GI tract. It is also reasonable to consider joint pain as part of another disease which may affect joints as well as blood vessels, as discussed below.

Astute blood laboratory technicians noticed that blood from patients with hepatitis C often developed a clump of insoluble material in the bottom of the tube when their blood was stored in a refrigerator for 1–3 days. This precipitate was identified as antibodies or immune proteins mixed with hepatitis C virus pieces. This protein precipitate, which appeared in the cold, was named "cryoglobulins." When careful tests are performed, *one of every three people infected with hepatitis C has serum cryoglobulins,* or antibodies bound to hepatitis C in the serum which precipitate (come out of solution or are no longer dissolved) when the serum is placed on ice.

What are cryoglobulins? They are complexes of hepatitis C bound to antibodies and other molecules from the immune system (rheumatoid factor, complement and immunoglobulins). These complexes circulate in the body and deposit in the small blood vessels in the kidneys, legs, and arms. When they wind up resting in these blood vessels, the complexes of hepatitis C and immune molecules cause injury or inflammation to the blood vessels (vasculitis).

Purpura or bruises can be one of the most easily recognized signs of vasculitis associated with cryoglobulinemia, which is the presence of cold-precipitable proteins in the blood. Cryoglobulins are detected by storing blood at 4°C for 24–72 hours and checking for a precipitate which can be seen with the eye. The cryoglobulin is composed of immune complexes of antibodies and hepatitis C antigens. Cryloglobulins may be detected after viral, bacterial or parasitic infections, rheumatologic disorders or lymphoma. The good news is that they usually go away after treatment of the primary disorder.

There used to be a large group of people who had chronic, relapsing bouts of joint aches, bruises, and weakness for whom an underlying disorder could not be readily identified. This unknown group was referred to as having essential mixed cryoglobulinemia, EMC for short. We now know that hepatitis C is its major cause, implicated in most if not all cases of EMC. While 1 out of 3 people infected with hepatitis C has cryoglobulins, only 1–2% of people with hepatitis C have essential mixed cryoglobulinemia. If people have not reached end-stage liver disease, they are often treated with interferon.

Vascular injury results from immune complex deposition leading to an actual attack of the immune system damaging vessel walls. One out of 4 people with essential mixed cryoglobulinemia also could develop glomerulonephritis, a disorder in which the part of the kidney responsible for filtering blood gets thickened deposits of immune complexes and can no longer do its job. It's like a drain in a shower getting plugged up by hair, only the hair in this case is hepatitis C antibody conjugates and the drain is the kidney. Male sex, older age at onset, severe proteinuria (protein in the urine), and bad kidney function all signal a worse outlook for this hepatitis C-associated kidney disease characterized by plugging of the renal filters, membranoproliferative glomerulonephritis.

The treatment of cryloglobulinemias is aimed at attacking the underlying cause, in this case, treating hepatitis C. Medicines may be used to ease symptoms, such as anti-inflammatory drugs which ease joint pain. Management of kidney dysfunction also includes dietary, fluid and serum salt management as well as maintenance on hemodialysis if necessary. Steroids, immunosuppressives, and plasmapheresis are sometimes attempted as treatments as well.

Hepatitis C is a virus which primarily infects the liver but also circulates at high concentrations in the blood. It may have effects outside the liver, including skin, joint, and blood vessel disease. There may also be an increase in some antibodies directed against parts of the individual's own body, so-called autoimmune antibodies. These antibodies are generally detected in low concentration, but may also occasionally appear in significant quantities, particularly against the thyroid gland. There appears to be a propensity for a small fraction of people infected with hepatitis C to develop inflammation of the thyroid gland, and this may be exacerbated by interferon treatment. In summary, while it is easy to focus on the direct effects of hepatitis C on the liver, a variety of other systemic signs of infection may be of equal or greater concern to the individual who suffers with the infection. It is therefore important to consider the impact of hepatitis C infection on the joints, kidneys, nerves, thyroid, and skin as well as other potential sites for active disease which may be further defined.

14

Hepatitis C and Your Kidneys

The normal function of the kidneys is to filter blood. They permit elimination of excess fluid and wastes in the urine, while allowing the body to retain important salts and elements. This process is tightly regulated so that levels of salts and fluids are maintained relatively constant in the body. Having a sick liver disrupts this balance and interferes with the normal functioning of the kidneys.

How do the kidneys contribute to the formation of ascites (the accumulation of fluid in the abdomen)? In the setting of end-stage liver disease, blood protein levels fall and fluid seeps out of blood vessels into the abdomen taking the form of ascites. The kidneys then perceive the blood volume as being too low, which triggers a response of avidly holding onto salt, even as the total quantity of salt present in the blood vessels and ascites or abdominal fluid may overload the body. The salt in turn causes the body to retain more fluid, further worsening ascites and potentially even decreasing urine output. For every gram of excess sodium which the body retains, 200 grams or more of water is retained. For this reason, people with end-stage liver disease are often advised to limit their intake of salt to 1 gram, which is the same as 1,000 mg of salt per day. To appreciate how little salt this entails, 1 teaspoon of table salt contains 2100 mg of salt.

Keeping to a salt-restricted diet is a herculean task which is made more difficult by years of habitual excess salt intake by some individuals. For starters, pitch the salt shaker off the table and into the garbage. No added salt at the time of meal preparation or once the plate hits the table. As people try to change their seasoning habits it is easy to run in to trouble with other spices or sauces high in salt. Soy sauce and teriyaki sauce are notoriously salt rich, as are garlic salt, bouillon, steak sauces, and many barbecue sauces.

Processed foods are frequently shockingly stocked with sodium. Some examples include a cup of chicken noodle soup which alone exceeds the limit at 1006 mg sodium, a bowl of cereal may contain 375 mg sodium, and red meats may be high in sodium as well. Frozen foods also can be high in salts, so careful reading of labels while shopping is a grand idea. Fast foods are another eye opener. Burger King's bacon double cheeseburger weighs in with 1220 mg salt. One of Arby's subs contains 1354 mg sodium, and that is before any dressing is added! Two slices of Domino's cheese pizza weigh in at 980 mg sodium. McDonald's quarter-pounder with cheese? It's got 1160 mg sodium. Wendy's big bacon classic, 1500 mg sodium. Home fries have 745 mg sodium. It is hard to order fast food low in sodium, but not impossible. For example, some salads without dressing may be low in salt. Burger King's apple pie tips the scales at only 30 mg sodium. Eating out in more tradi-tional restaurants is a big challenge, too. Professional chefs use a lot more salt than you might imagine, so judicious order-ing of items cooked specifically to be low in salt is the best bet. Again, be cautious of prepared soups, which almost always are laden with sodium.

What if you cook at home, what common foods are high in salt? Many processed meats are laden with salt, particularly

Table 10. Foods with Low
Levels of Salt

Fresh fruit	0 mg
Vegetables, unsalted	0 mg
Pasta, unsalted	10 mg/serving
Rice, unsalted	10 mg/serving
Fish or chicken, unsalted	30 mg/ounce
Soup, low-salt	20 mg/serving
Ice cream, gelatin, low-salt	50 mg/serving

ham, bacon, sausage, corned beef, smoked or cured meats, and sliced sandwich meats like bologna or roast beef. Some dairy products have more salt than others. Buttermilk, for example, is much higher in salt than skim milk. Most cheeses, particularly processed cheeses and cottage cheese, are also high in salt. Vegetables are usually low in salt unless they are canned with salt or pickled. Vegetable juices also may have high salt content, as can olives, sauerkraut, and relish. Frozen pasta and rice dishes have often been boiled with salt. Many ready-made foods, like potato chips, peanuts, pretzels, and tortilla chips are also often loaded with salt. Breakfast cereals, including precooked hot cereals, may also have quite a bit of salt. Not all foods are high in salt; read product labels carefully, paying attention to the salt or sodium chloride concentration per serving.

One pitfall: People who are observant of their blood tests may think that they do not have enough salt if they notice their serum sodium is low. In other words, if normal serum sodium concentrations are 138 (mEq/L), and someone with ascites has a sodium concentration of 120 (mEq/L), this does not mean they need to consume more salt. Nor does it mean that they don't have to bother with a salt restriction. People with ascites are almost always overloaded with salt in terms of their total body salt, including the salt in the ascites. The serum sodium concentration may fall as a result of dilution of the sodium from excessive retained fluid. The absolute amount of total body sodium is often still too high, so this is treated with salt and fluid restrictions. It is best to discuss salt and fluid restrictions with a physician rather than attempting to set a course of treatment on your own.

Fortunately, patients with hepatitis C who are not troubled by ascites may eat a diet with prudent salt content without adhering to a strict sodium restriction. Consistently watching what you eat is instrumental to maintaining good health if you have problems with ascites. If you have ascites, one focus of your diet should be to lower the amount of fluid retained in your abdomen, and that translates into controlling sodium and water intake.

Hepatitis C-infected people with liver disease complicated by ascites or fluid retention have kidneys that simply cannot get rid of the excess salt accumulating in their body the way the way the kidneys normally would. The accumulation of salt carries with it the accumulation of fluid. In addition to dietary discretion, this kidney dysfunction in the setting of liver disease is routinely treated with diuretics, drugs that make people urinate. The most effective regimens involve combinations of the drugs furosemide (Lasix) along with spironolactone (Aldactone) or amiloride (Midamor). Use of these drugs requires careful monitoring of serum salt concentrations, as serum sodium and potassium levels can fluctuate over time with these drugs, particularly in the setting of severe liver disease.

As liver disease progresses over time, the degree of kidney dysfunction may worsen considerably. Initially, this may be manifest as an inability to regulate fluids and electrolytes as well as in the past, which then requires more frequent paracentesis procedures to drain ascitic fluid from the abdomen, as in the case of Rudy. It may also require more aggressive restrictions on the intake of salt and fluid. Not only is it important to exclude sodium chloride (NaCl) from the diet, but it is also important to avoid some salt substitutes which may contain large quantities of equally troublesome potassium chloride (KCl). Naturally, as salt intake is restricted and diuretics are used to make people urinate more, they become thirstier. If people with end-stage liver disease drink excessive quantities of fluid, it can defeat the purpose of using diuretics and salt restriction. It is therefore best to monitor fluid intake and bring excessive consumption (more than 1–2 L/day) to the attention of a physician.

The most severe state of renal dysfunction in the setting of end-stage liver disease is known as hepatorenal syndrome, in which the kidneys respond to a failing liver by failing themselves. This condition of dynamic imbalance has a grim prognosis. The hepatorenal syndrome is diagnosed by excluding other causes of renal failure. Characteristics of hepatorenal syndrome include a rising concentration of serum proteins normally eliminated through the kidneys, urea and creatinine, along with a drop in urine production in the setting of a normal urine sediment (analysis of the urine for signs of infection, obstruction or other kidney diseases), adequate hydration and a low output of sodium in the urine. Once hepatorenal syndrome has progressed too severely, options include confronting the futility of the situation (admitting nature will take its course) or liver transplantation along with renal transplantation. Kidney dialysis alone is rarely used unless liver transplantation is anticipated at some point in the future. The best way to prevent hepatorenal syndrome is to take care of your liver and avoid end-stage liver disease. This is one of the reasons efforts are made to treat hepatitis C infection with interferon-containing regimens. Once end-stage liver disease sets in, hepatorenal syndrome may be forestalled by maintaining careful control of the dietary salt and fluid intake, as well as regular physician visits to monitor serum sodium and potassium levels, fluid status, and kidney and liver function.

There are other renal diseases which may affect a subset of hepatitis C-infected individuals even before the onset of end-stage liver disease. The body makes antibodies in response to hepatitis C infection. Following an acute infection, these antibodies can actually be quite plentiful, but unfortunately they do not clear the virus from the body in most cases.

They may circulate in the person's serum bound to the virus coat and may even lead to deposition of antibodies bound to viruses throughout the body. When these complexes deposit in blood vessel walls they can lead to inflammation of the blood vessels (vasculitis). When they deposit in the skin these antibodies bound to viruses (viral antigen antibody complexes) can lead to inflammation of the skin's blood vessels, which makes bruises. Very frequently they can also be filtered from the blood to be deposited in the kidneys, causing renal disease. One common form of kidney disease which is seen with hepatitis C has the long name membranoproliferative glomerulonephritis, a disease in which the cellular filters in the kidney become plugged up.

Another common form of kidney disease seen in people with liver disease is called "IgA nephropathy," which is another disease where the kidneys get clogged up. IgA nephropathy probably results from failure of the diseased liver to filter or remove excess or old immunoglobulins from the blood. Normally Kupffer cells, one of the types of cells in the liver, suck up IgA which is circulating in the blood to get rid of leftover or old IgA which is no longer needed. As the liver becomes sick, the Kupffer cells no longer perform this critical function and immunoglobin proteins then build up in the blood. If the process gets too severe, then circulating immunoglobins can be deposited in the kidneys. If these deposits become excessive, kidney function may fail. The condition is suggested by high serum IgA levels and confirmed by renal biopsy. Renal biopsy consists of removing a small core of kidney tissue and looking at it under a microscope. These kidney diseases can occur at any time during hepatitis C infection but become more likely as the disease progresses.

The best way to prevent these kidney diseases from occurring is to clear the virus from the person's circulation with antiviral treatments such as interferon. Several studies have documented improvement in glomerulonephritis in response to interferon treatment of hepatitis C infection. Unfortunately, not all people with hepatitis C-induced glomerulonephritis can tolerate or respond to interferon treatment.

The kidneys play a critical role in regulating salt and fluid levels in the body. As liver disease progresses, these critical kidney functions cease to work automatically. In essence, it is necessary to consciously monitor your fluid and salt intake to keep your body in good balance. Careful dietary control along with diuretic treatment can help manage some of the disparities caused by deteriorating kidney function. Several renal diseases associated with hepatitis C infection, such as IgA nephropathy and glomerulonephritis, may be treated or prevented by addressing the underlying hepatitis C infection.

15

Your Immune System

Approximately 40% of those infected with the human immunodeficiency virus (HIV), which causes AIDS, are also infected with hepatitis C. This high concordance of infection may well be a result of common risk factors for the spread of both diseases. Alternatively, people with HIV infection may be more susceptible to infection with hepatitis C. Certainly we know that hepatitis C virus is even more common than HIV in the population of the United States, and therefore the probability of acquiring hepatitis C is high among individuals who use intravenous drugs, who received blood transfusions before 1992 or who engage in high-risk practices wherein exposure to blood or blood products is likely.

Since the hepatitis C virus infects people with HIV, one critical question is whether the disease follows the same course in individuals infected with both HIV and hepatitis C as in those infected with hepatitis C alone. This is an area of intensive focus, because it appears that the hepatitis C virus runs a more aggressive course in the immunosuppressed person—e.g., someone infected with HIV. It is important to note that numerous treatments that have been tried for people infected with both hepatitis C and HIV have not shown substantial benefit. The viral protease inhibitors that are highly effective in keeping HIV in check for a while do not appear to have any significant activity against the hepatitis C virus. In addition, the agents such as interferon that appear to be beneficial in the treatment of some hepatitis C-infected individuals do not appear to work as well in people infected with hepatitis C and HIV. Interferon is used to treat Kaposi's sarcoma in AIDS patients, but this is a form of cancer associated with AIDS. Interferon is not used to fight the HIV virus itself. The fact that interferon does not work as well against hepatitis C in immunocompromised people is not surprising. Interferon stimulates the immune system to fight the hepatitis C virus rather than having a direct antiviral effect on hepatitis C in particular.

The effects of interferon treatment on hepatitis C in the immunocompromised individual have been studied; unfortunately, the few clinical trials to date have demonstrated substantial lowering of interferon's effectiveness against HCV in patients coinfected with HCV and HIV. Whether there will be subsets of HIV-infected persons, perhaps those who do not demonstrate evidence of HIV disease on blood tests (normal CD4 counts), is one area for further study and hope. Perhaps these individuals will continue to respond to interferon or other combination hepatitis C treatments. Certainly people coinfected with hepatitis C and HIV would like to treat their hepatitis C, but the best way to do this is not known. Since all of these antiviral drugs have toxicities, perhaps it may be best to treat coinfected individuals in controlled clinical trials, given the unclear benefit of potentially toxic drugs in treating the hepatitis C virus in the HIV-infected individual.

Another question that comes up is the utility of liver transplantation in the individual coinfected with hepatitis C and HIV who suffers from end-stage liver disease. Several small clinical studies addressing this question have shown that HIV infection greatly exacerbates complications in liver transplant recipients. This may be due to the combination of posttransplant immunosuppression (to prevent organ rejection) and HIV infection, or to more rapid progression of hepatitis C reinfection of the liver graft. Most of these small studies were done before protease inhibitors were available to control HIV infection, and therefore people infected with both who receive liver transplantation may fare better now than they would have in the past. Perhaps these people would best be treated in the setting of a well-performed clinical trial, to get a clearer answer to the question of HIV infection's impact on the course of hepatitis C infection in individuals after their liver transplant. This could benefit not only the people enrolled in the study, but also other individuals who suffer from similar ailments.

People coinfected with HIV and hepatitis C seem to experience a more rapid course in their hepatitis C infection, which raises the question as to whether other forms of immunosuppression (such as use of immunosuppressant medications) or other immune deficiency states (such as diabetes or other congenital immune deficiency syndromes) may trigger a more aggressive course of hepatitis C infection. The evidence from liver transplantation in the hepatitis C-infected individual suggests that hepatitis C runs a more aggressive course in the immunosuppressed patient. Following individuals placed on prednisone, cyclosporine, and immuran after transplant, the use of immunosuppressive drugs revealed that most people actively infected with circulating hepatitis C virus prior to transplantation reinfect their liver graft. There are a number of studies in progress to see if this can be prevented or treated, and it is likely that people with hepatitis C will be treated to decrease or diminish the probability of hepatitis C reinfection of the new liver. Treatment regimens are likely to include drugs such as interferon and ribavirin, as well as hepatitis C viral protease inhibitors, as they become available.

We know that people with hepatitis C who receive liver transplants do get the infection back in their new liver. They progress to cirrhosis of the liver within approximately 5–7 years of their transplant. Fortunately, most of these liver transplant recipients maintain good liver function and may add decades to their lives by receiving a liver transplant. Remember, it usually took decades for hepatitis C to scar over their original liver, and many people live with a scarred-over or cirrhotic liver for many more years before decompensated liver disease develops. After liver transplantation, some people run this course even more quickly, and it is not unusual for individuals to have cirrhosis in the donated graft as early as 6 months after transplantation. We also know that people who get infected when they are older, such as people who contract hepatitis C at the time of coronary artery bypass grafting, tend to have a more aggressive course of hepatitis C infection than those who contract the virus at a younger age. Once again, this may be due to a weakened immune system in an elderly person in comparison to a younger one. Alternatively it may be due to preexisting damage in the older liver, which is unable to mount an effective regenerative response to infection.

16

Psychological Impact of Hepatitis C

Jack walked into the clinic. He said, "I can't take it anymore; I can't even put a worm on a fishhook." He was shaking and trembling. "I'm just not myself anymore. I feel anxious all the time. My hands don't work right. I feel sweaty on my forehead and in the palms of my hands just sitting in a chair. Sometimes I think I will kill myself."

Dr. Bates gazed at him. To assess how serious he was, he asked, "Have you thought about how you would kill yourself?"

"I want to take a shotgun and blow my head off. I've been thinking I should remove all the guns from my house."

Dr. Bates asked him, "Have you ever tried to kill yourself?"

"Yes, once when I was drunk I put my head into a hot convection oven, but then the phone rang so I had to answer it."

At this point Dr. Bates felt that the patient needed the help of a psychiatrist. He picked up the phone, called, and had the patient seen promptly.

Hepatitis C can exact an enormous emotional toll on its victims. Quite often the emotional signs are much more subtle and harder to correlate directly with the infection than in Jack's case. It is not that hepatitis C is believed to directly affect the central nervous system, but because of the diverse effects it has on the body, it certainly can influence one's psyche. As people lose energy, they may not feel like interacting with others. They may not be up to pursuing their usual activities. When suffering from joint aches and pains, they may not feel capable of operating athletic equipment, performing manual labor, carrying out everyday chores, or engaging in other activities essential to professional or social interaction. Thus hepatitis C's debilitating symptoms can have a substantial psychosocial impact on one's life. Furthermore, by rendering a person into a couch potato, it chips away at one's sense of self-worth.

The diagnosis of hepatitis C can reduce one's self-esteem. Friends and even family may avoid the hepatitis C-infected individual out of irrational fear of contracting the disease. Neither of these needs to happen, so it is important that the disease be properly understood. Since the disease is quite prevalent in society, the infected individual does not have to feel that he is alone; *1 out of 50 people in this country is infected.*

The news that one is infected with hepatitis C virus can have a variable impact on different individuals. Because hepatitis C has many different faces, the diagnosis of hepatitis C carries different importance to different people. Many people deal with the diagnosis simply through denial. If they feel fine, it is hard for them to grapple with the potential threat to life that the virus imposes and the infectious risk it poses to others. On the other hand, hepatitis C infection may emotionally devastate individuals knowing the potential seriousness of the diagnosis. In many cases, the illness may be psychologically dealt with much like other chronic illnesses, such as diabetes or hypertension. There may be feelings of guilt if the infection was obtained through intravenous drug use or sexual contact.

But most of all, as mentioned previously, there also may be feelings of diminished self-worth. People may feel contaminated and too enervated to work. Part of the difficulty in grappling with the emotional issues that go along with hepatitis C infection is dealing with the uncertainty that goes along with the diagnosis. Since the illness takes different courses in different people, it is easy for the individual to overreact to the diagnosis. Someone with a mild, early case of the disease may feel like they are dying, when this could not be further from the truth. Similarly, someone with advanced disease may use the variable disease course as license to deny the importance of his or her particular prognosis. Finally, not knowing the exact course your hepatitis C infection will take, having to live with uncertainty can crank up the anxiety.

The diagnosis of hepatitis C may have devastating consequences. It may come when an individual is having decompensated liver disease, and an urgent transplant workup may be necessary. It may come when liver transplantation is impracticable, and may actually be an explanation for why someone is dying. Alternatively it may come when a person has no symptoms, is highly functional and working and doesn't feel any impact whatsoever of the viral infection.

Similarly, the diagnosis may come as a surprise for individuals who have limited or mild symptoms and may proceed with the virus for 60 or 70 years with no untoward effects. On the other hand, people with minimal symptoms may progress rapidly to end-stage liver disease in the short term. For these reasons, coping with the diagnosis of hepatitis C can be extremely difficult. As stated previously, the uncertainty involved with the diagnosis and its impact on the person's health can also cause a great deal of anxiety. Some anxiety may be relieved by a medical evaluation and counseling, or even a liver biopsy to evaluate the state of the liver at the time in which the diagnosis is made. Others may choose to deal with the problem through denial, in effect assuming that they will be one of the lucky ones whom the virus will not strike. This approach is recklessly inappropriate. With the emergence of improved treatment techniques, it is realistic to expect that some people with hepatitis C virus may now be routinely cured. Therefore it is imperative that hepatitis C-infected individuals be evaluated to determine whether they elect to undergo treatment with current regimens, enroll in experimental protocols to test theoretically improved regimens or defer treatment and undergo close medical observation every 6–12 months until such time as their condition changes or new treatments develop.

Hepatitis C infection also can place tremendous strains on family and friends. Obviously if a person has shared recreational drugs with others, he may be infected. Certainly, it may be beneficial to test for the virus in sexual contacts as well. If a person is involved in a monogamous relationship, this also may pose a tremendous strain on that relationship because the diagnosis may carry with it the potential that one of the two partners may have given the virus to the other. Maybe there was infidelity. Certainly it is prudent for people to be checked for infection. In addition there is a small but real risk of transmission from mother to child. The diagnosis in a mother may therefore implicate hepatitis C infection on her children (a small risk). All of these concerns need to be addressed directly; not discussing them can create even greater anxiety.

With the growing knowledge about hepatitis C infection, hepatitis C-infected individuals are able to get clear answers and a better understanding of the impact of the virus on their lives. How each person deals with that information, however, can vary. One unfortunate aspect of medical care is the physician's limited time with patients. Office visits tend to focus on treatment of medical symptoms and direct viral toxicity and less on the emotional impact of viral infection. Alternative sources of support include clinic nurses, friends, or relatives who may also be infected and support groups. Patient support groups can be a helpful way for people to share the problems that the virus has caused them and their emotional upsets with other people who have similar problems. There are growing networks of support groups throughout the country with many choices present in most major cities.

Nevertheless, everyone must deal with the diagnosis in his own way and it is important for physicians, as well as patients, to be attuned to potential depression which may result from the diagnosis. Of course, not everyone with hepatitis C infection is disabled, nor should everyone view themselves that way. Many individuals are able to go on with work and enjoy healthy, productive lives for many decades while carrying the diagnosis. It may be difficult for these patients to confront the need for treatment at this time.

Treatment can bring on stresses of its own. Individuals may defer life decisions, job assignments or family commitments because they feel overwhelmed by the burden of treatment. An added stress of viral infection may be caused by treatment methods, some of which (such as interferon) can affect mood, triggering anxiety or depression. All of these emotional effects must be kept in mind throughout the course of the hepatitis C infection. The burden of having a chronic medical illness such as hepatitis C infection must be dealt with until the virus is cured.

It is reasonable for individuals with hepatitis C infection to seek counseling from social workers, psychiatrists, psychologists, or religious leaders. This can be difficult if these healthcare providers and advisers are not familiar with hepatitis C. Therefore, obtaining counseling from someone who understands the many different manifestations of viral infection and understands the impact of the virus on the individual's health is best. Counselors with this expertise may be found by referral from a hepatologist, or liver specialist.

Finally, it is important to recognize that a number of individuals with hepatitis C infection have a problem with alcohol that they may not want to admit. Even mild alcohol consumption may pose a risk to individuals infected with hepatitis C, and everyone infected with hepatitis C needs to come to grips with this possibility. It is crucial to recognize that the diagnosis of hepatitis C may lead some people to drink more, since alcohol may be a stress or anxiety coping mechanism for some people. Because alcohol intake could be disastrous to their health, appropriate referral to Alcoholics Anonymous or alcohol rehab may be prudent. Alcoholism is a frequent comorbid condition with hepatitis C infection, and there may be other comorbid illnesses such as hepatitis B infection, HIV infection, or other problems to which healthcare providers should be attuned.

The best way for an individual to deal with the diagnosis of hepatitis C infection is to seek appropriate medical attention and become educated about his or her own health and disease. Only when people are thus empowered can they obtain appropriate follow-up. Certainly a sense of effectively managing one's disease can do much to relieve anxiety and prevent detrimental psychological and social impacts from the disease. Many people do not tell their friends that they are infected, because they fear being stigmatized. However, the infected person and his or her sexual partner should take precautions, particularly if one has multiple sexual partners. Certainly there is no reason for someone with hepatitis C to be stigmatized, and yet concern, unfortunately, may not be unfounded, because the general population needs to be better educated about this disease. It is not uncommon for an individual to avoid talking about the infection with anyone. This certainly can lead to increased anxiety, as well as generate misunderstanding about the infection or about the person's own health status. Certainly an improved understanding, not only for individuals infected with hepatitis C but also for insurers, employers and society as a whole, will lead to greater support for people affected with this debilitating disease.

Lack of adequate financial support is an unfortunate reality for most people infected with hepatitis C. The cost of physician visits, medicines, and time lost from work can all mount to generate havoc with an individual's budget. The treatments themselves may decrease energy and productivity as they attempt to rid the body of its viral invader. Having financial problems but being reluctant to discuss the reason can lead to even further anxiety and stress. It is easy to blame lack of ambition or success on a disease that is known to instigate fatigue, generating a poor attitude which may predispose one to failure. The process of seeking financial help can seem daunting.

FINANCIAL IMPACT OF THE DISEASE

In our capitalist society, goods are rationed on the basis of financial means. Unfortunately, treating health care as a commodity carries with it the peril that not everyone may be able to afford it. This book has discussed a broad range of treatment and screening options, but not every infected individual may have access to these without some assistance. While most health insurance companies cover treatments for hepatitis C, not surprisingly some restrict access to specialists or medicines. Note that most of these payment systems have appeal mechanisms, and the infected individual should feel comfortable challenging denial of treatment if his physician feels it is indicated. Alarmingly, close to 1 in 5 Americans is not covered by health insurance, so they may not even be able to see a physician to address their questions. Certainly, infected individuals need access to medical care and should maintain health insurance if at all possible.

There are also numerous avenues of public assistance available to those who need it. Unfortunately, it can require diligence to navigate the bureaucratic maze to enroll in public assistance programs such as Medicaid. Pharmaceutical programs have also set aside allotments for relief medicines for the indigent. The best way to access these systems is with the help of a hospital or physician. For those with advanced liver disease, Social Security disability may also be available; infected individuals frequently get the help of an attorney in filing the necessary paperwork to enroll in these programs. Local social workers can be a good source of advice for how best to ask for financial help, considering the financial hit hepatitis C can take on the un- or underinsured.

The financial impact of hepatitis C is easy to underestimate. Besides direct medical bills, individuals may suffer from lost work time, sick days, decreased productivity, an increased need for help with childcare responsibilities or an increased need for home healthcare assistance. People can lose their jobs if their performance lags, and if they do not know they are infected with hepatitis C they may not even know why their energy has failed. Obviously the need for attentive medical diagnosis and care can become more difficult for individuals with compromised finances. If there is a history of military service, Veterans Administration Medical Centers may be another resource for healthcare and support.

17

Epilogue

The prospect of being infected with hepatitis C is truly frightening, but must be carefully tempered by the reality that a percentage of infected individuals may not be strongly adversely affected for some time. The incubation period, or time of symptom-free infection, varies from one individual to another, but may be many decades long. Unfortunately, of the 4 million infected Americans, the majority have already been infected for a number of decades.

As we learn more about the hepatitis C virus, new treatments are being developed which are more effective at eliminating the virus from infected individuals. Similarly, as we study people who are infected, we are learning that environmental factors, such as alcohol use, greatly speed up the pace with which hepatitis C ravages the liver. New treatments will be able to cure more people of the hepatitis C virus, and new knowledge is already enabling others to slow down the disease course in their bodies.

With the large number of symptom-free hepatitis C-infected people now progressing toward cirrhosis, unless more aggressive efforts are made to treat and cure this infection, the number of deaths from hepatitis C will triple over the next decade.

To put this into perspective, think of everyone you know who has suffered from breast cancer. Forty thousand people die from breast cancer every year; in a decade the number of people dying from hepatitis C complications may be only slightly less. *As noted, we now know that alcohol greatly accelerates the injury from this virus, so hepatitis C-infected individuals should refrain from drinking.* Other measures, such as following a healthy diet and maintaining good liver health, may slow the rate of progression.

Fortunately, the government, private foundations, and physicians are responding to the hepatitis C challenge with more aggressive efforts to educate and treat infected individuals. More important, infected individuals are actively seeking out help to control or rid themselves of this infection. Only when infected people are fully empowered to fight this long-term problem can hepatitis C be conquered.

The era in which this disease was ignored or its effects were denied has passed quickly. It is important that denial not be replaced with hysteria. Some recent TV news reports have pictured long faces with statements comparing hepatitis C to AIDS. There are important differences. At least a fraction of hepatitis C patients can be cured with present treatments. The hepatitis C virus has a much longer symptom-free period than HIV in most cases, and many infected people may not develop severe symptoms. Finally, it is harder to transmit the hepatitis C virus through sexual exposure, so it may well be easier to control the spread of this virus now that good tests are available to detect tainted blood. Advances in curtailing intravenous drug abuse as well as developing safer, more sterile practices such as needle exchange programs for those who continue to abuse drugs are needed. The most common defined route of spread for new hepatitis C infections today is intravenous drug use. Infected individuals, particularly those who have had multiple partners, can use barrier contraception with sexual partners to be safest. Contact with hepatitis C-infected blood needs to be avoided.

Many challenges remain before hepatitis C is fully conquered. These include developing a vaccine for the virus, improving treatments so that the majority of infected individuals are cured, and doing a better job of screening exposed and at-risk individuals for hepatitis C infection. *As many as 9 out of 10 infected individuals do not know they harbor the disease; they need to be diagnosed.* Once diagnosed, they may consider treatment, lifestyle modification, and reduce the risk of spread of the disease. Present treatments involving interferon and ribavirin, though hopeful, entail substantial risks of side effects, so improvements in treatment effectiveness and safety are still needed.

It is important that people infected with hepatitis C not feel stigmatized or alone. Since the virus infects 1 in 50 Americans, the infected individual probably has company in any modest-size group. Hepatitis C is not spread by laughing, singing, hugging, kissing, coughing, or casual contact. There is no reason to exclude infected individuals from social, educational, or occupational functions. While such exclusion is a common fear of infected individuals, fortunately this kind of fear-fueled discrimination has yet to be a major problem.

One of the most important steps that need to be taken is to screen individuals at risk for infection because of their exposure history or because of prior high-risk behavior such as even just once experimenting with intravenous drugs or intranasal cocaine. Since there is a long symptomless incubation period, it is necessary to discover who is infected so that we may stem the spread of disease. We also need to know who is infected so that people can be offered treatment both now and in the future, as even better treatments become available. Other coexisting liver illnesses that may accelerate the rate of progression of liver disease also must be ascertained and treated. Further research on the natural course of hepatitis C infection is needed.

As people develop end-stage liver disease complicated by confusion, bleeding, abdominal fluid collections (ascites), or muscle wasting, they need to consider liver transplantation as an option to potentially prolong their life. Care for patients with severe liver disease has improved greatly, and medical and certain shunt treatments may also prolong people's lives in the future. Once someone has cirrhosis from hepatitis C, there is up to a 3% annual risk of developing a liver cancer. These cancers can be difficult to detect and treat, so how best to screen for and treat liver cancers is another topic which warrants future research.

Greater resources need to be brought to bear to address the growing shortage of donor liver organs. Hepatitis C is the leading cause of end-stage liver disease as a precipitating cause of liver transplantation, and we need to make every effort to ensure that any potential organ donor is offered the option of passing their healthy liver on to someone with a critical, life-or-death need. Better treatments to prevent reinfection with hepatitis C after liver transplant are also necessary.

The future holds many challenges both for the individuals infected with hepatitis C and for those who try to help them. The pace of advances in hepatitis C knowledge will no doubt continue to be rapid. The techniques of molecular biology and genetics which have increased our knowledge of cancer, heart disease, and diabetes are also augmenting our understanding of liver diseases. Technology is driving discovery at a rapid pace. Since hepatitis C was discovered less than a decade ago, it is remarkable that we are already able to cure 20–40% of infected individuals in selected patient populations enrolled in clinical trials. It is hard to believe that the pace of discovery will not be even more rapid over the next decade.

Bibliography

Chapters 1, Introduction to the Illness; 2, Discovering Hepatitis C

1. National Institutes of Health. 1997. Consensus development conference panel statement: management of hepatitis C. *Hepatology* 26(3)(suppl 1): 2S–10S.
2. Bacon BR. 1997. Iron and hepatitis C. *Gut* 41:127–128.
3. Shimizu, YK, H Igarashi, T Kiyohara, M Shapiro, DC Wong, RH Purcell, and H Yoshikura. 1998. Infection of a chimpanzee with hepatitis C virus grown in cell culture. *J Gen Virol* 79:1383–1386.
4. Shiffman ML. 1998. Management of hepatitis C. DDW prototype. *Clin Perspect Gastroenterol* 6–19.
5. Lee AU, GC Farrell. 1997. Drug-induced liver disease. *Curr Opin Gastroenterol* 13:199–205.
6. Jenny-Avital ER. 1998. Hepatitis C. *Curr Opin Infect Dis* 11:293–299.
7. Yanagi M, M St. Claire, M Shapiro, SU Emerson, RH Purcell, J Bukh. 1998. Transcripts of a chimeric cDNA clone of hepatitis C virus genotype 1b are infectious in vivo. *Virology* 244:161–172.
8. Major ME, SM Feinstone. 1997. The molecular virology of hepatitis C. *Hepatology* 25:1527–1538.
9. Purcell R. 1997. The hepatitis C virus: overview. *Hepatology* 26(suppl 1): 11S–14S.
10. Hoofnagle JH. 1997. Hepatitis C: the clinical spectrum of disease. *Hepatology* 26(suppl 1):15S–20S.
11. Witte DL. 1997. Mild liver enzyme abnormalities: eliminating hemochromatosis as cause. *Clin Chem* 43:1535–1538.

12. Hoofnagle JH, TS Tralka. 1997. The National Institutes of Health consensus development conference: management of hepatitis C—Introduction. *Hepatology* 26(suppl 1):1S.
13. Diepolder HM, R Zachoval, RM Hoffmann, EA Wierenga, T Santantonio, MC Jung, D Eichenlaub, GR Pape. 1995. Possible mechanism involving T-lymphocyte response to non-structural protein 3 in viral clearance in acute hepatitis C virus infection. *Lancet* 346:1006–1007.
14. Choo QL, G Kuo, A Weiner, et al. 1992. Identification of the major, parenteral non-A non-B hepatitis agent (hepatitis C virus) using a recombinant approach. *Semin Liver Dis* 12:279–288.
15. Choo QL, KH Richman, JH Han, K Berger, C Lee, C Dong, et al. 1991. Genetic organization and diversity of the hepatitis C virus. *Proc Natl Acad Sci USA* 88:2451–2455.
16. Houghton M, A Weiner, J Han, G Kuo, QL Choo. 1991. Molecular biology of the hepatitis C viruses: implications for diagnosis and control of viral disease. *Hepatology* 14(2):381–388.
17. Bukh J, RH Purcell, RH Miller. 1994. Sequence analysis of the core gene of 14 hepatitis C virus genotypes. *Proc Natl Acad Sci USA* 91:8239–8243.
18. Yanagi M, RH Purcell, SU Emerson, J Bukh. 1997. Transcripts from a single full-length cDNA clone of hepatitis C virus are infectious when directly transfected into the liver of a chimpanzee. *Proc Natl Acad Sci USA* 94:8738–8743.
19. Clarke B. 1997. Molecular virology of hepatitis C virus. *J Gen Virol* 78:2397–2410.
20. Neville JA, LE Prescott, V Bhattacherjee, N Adams, I Pike, B Rodgers, A El-Zayadi, S Hamid, GM Dusheiko, AA Saeed, GH Haydon, P Simmonds. 1997. Antigenic variation of core, NS3, and NS5 proteins among genotypes of hepatitis C virus. *J Clin Microbiol* 35:3062–3070.
21. Seipp S, HM Mueller, E Pfaff, W Stremmel, L Theilmann, T Goeser. 1997. Establishment of persistent hepatitis C virus infection and replication in vitro. *J Gen Virol* 78:2467–2476.
22. Kwong AD. 1997. Hepatitis C virus NS3/4A protease. *Curr Opin Infect Dis* 10:485–490.
23. Hezode C, C Cazeneuve, O Coué, JM Pawlotsky, ES Zafrani, S Amselem, D Dhumeaux. 1998. Hemochromatosis Cys282Tyr mutation and liver iron overload in patients with chronic active hepatitis C. *Hepatology* 27:306.
24. McDonnell WM, FK Askari. 1997. Immunization. *JAMA* 278:2000–2007.
25. Tsarev SA, TS Tsareva, SU Emerson, S Govindarajan, M Shapiro, JL Gerin, RH Purcell. 1997. Recombinant vaccine against hepatitis E: dose response and protection against heterologous challenge. *Vaccine* 15:1834–1838.
26. Buratti E, M Gerotto, P Pontisso, A Alberti, SG Tisminetzky, FE Baralle. 1997. In vivo translational efficiency of different hepatitis C virus 5'-UTRs. *FEBS Lett* 411:275–280.

27. Neddermann P, L Tomei, C Steinkühler, P Gallinari, A Tramontano, R De Francesco. 1997. The nonstructural proteins of the hepatitis C virus: structure and functions. *Biol Chem Hoppe Seyler* 378:469–476.
28. Tafi R, R Bandi, C Prezzi, MU Mondelli, R Cortese, P Monaci, A Nicosia. 1997. Identification of hepatitis C core mimotopes: improved methods for the selection and use of disease-related phage-displayed peptides. *Biol Chem Hoppe Seyler* 378:495–502.
29. Reed KE, CM Rice. 1998. Molecular characterization of hepatitis C virus. *Curr Stud Hematol Blood Transfus* 62:1–37.
30. Yuan ZH, U Kumar, HC Thomas, YM Wen, J Monjardino. 1997. Expression, purification, and partial characterization of hepatitis C RNA polymerase. *Biochem Biophys Res Commun* 232:231–235.
31. Inchauspe G, ME Major, I Nakano, L Vivitski, M Maisonnas, C Trépo. 1998. Immune responses against hepatitis C virus structural proteins following genetic immunisation. *Dev Biol Stand* 92:163–168.

Chapter 3, Hepatitis C and Chronic Hepatitis

1. National Institutes of Health. 1997. Consensus development conference panel statement: management of hepatitis C. *Hepatology* 26(3)(suppl 1): 2S–10S.
2. Berenguer M, TL Wright. 1998. Is the hepatocyte a Trojan horse for hepatitis C virus? *Gut* 42:456–458.
3. Shiffman ML. 1998. Management of hepatitis C. DDW Prototype. *Clin Perspect Gastroenterol* 6–19.
4. Zhu NL, A Khoshnan, R Schneider, M Matsumoto, G Dennert, C Ware, MMC Lai. 1998. Hepatitis C virus core protein binds to the cytoplasmic domain of tumor necrosis factor (TNF) receptor 1 and enhances TNF-induced apoptosis. *J Virol* 72:3691–3697.
5. Halsey NA, JS Abramson, PJ Chesney, MC Fisher, MA Gerber, DS Gromisch, S Kohl, SM Marcy, DL Murray, GD Overturf, RJ Whitley, R Yogev, G Peter, CB Hall, M Alter, B Schwartz, R Breiman, MC Hardegree, RF Jacobs, NE MacDonald, WA Orenstein, NR Rabinovich. 1998. Hepatitis C virus infection. *Pediatrics* 101:481–485.
6. Bassett SE, KM Brasky, RE Lanford. 1998. Analysis of hepatitis C virus–inoculated chimpanzees reveals unexpected clinical profiles. *J Virol* 72: 2589–2599.
7. Chang J, SH Yang, YG Cho, SB Hwang, YS Hahn, YC Sung. 1998. Hepatitis C virus core from two different genotypes has an oncogenic potential but is not sufficient for transforming primary rat embryo fibroblasts in cooperation with the H-*ras* oncogene. *J Virol* 72:3060–3065.
8. Thiele DL. 1997. Liver injury associated with hepatitis C infection: is it the virus or is it the host? Comments. *Hepatology* 26:238–239.

9. Schmidt WN, P Wu, J Cederna, FA Mitros, DR LaBrecque, JT Stapleton. 1997. Surreptitious hepatitis C virus (HCV) infection detected in the majority of patients with cryptogenic chronic hepatitis and negative hepatitis C antibody tests. *J Infect Dis* 176:27–33.

10. Ruggieri A, T Harada, Y Matsuura, T Miyamura. 1997. Sensitization to Fas-mediated apoptosis by hepatitis C virus core protein. *Virology* 229:68–76.

11. Marinella MA, RH Moseley. 1997. Hepatitis C and cancer. *Ann Intern Med* 126:1002–1003.

12. Takahashi M, G Yamada, R Miyamoto, T Doi, H Endo, T Tsuji. 1993. Natural course of chronic hepatitis C. *Am J Gastroenterol* 88:240–243.

13. Hoofnagle JH. 1997. Hepatitis C: the clinical spectrum of disease. *Hepatology* 26(suppl. 1):15S–20S.

14. Alter MJ, HS Margolis, K Krawczynski, et al. 1992. The natural history of community acquired hepatitis C in the United States. *N Engl J Med* 327:1899–1905.

15. Alter MJ. 1993. The detection, transmission, and outcome of hepatitis C infection. *Infect Agents Dis* 2:155–166.

16. Shimizu YK, M Hijikata, A Iwamoto, et al. 1994. Neutralizing antibodies against hepatitis C virus and the emergence of neutralization escape mutant viruses. *J Virol* 68:1494–1500.

17. Shirai M, T Akatsuka, CD Pendleton, R Houghten, C Wychowski, K Mihalik, S Feinstone, JA Berzofsky. 1992. Induction of cytotoxic T cells to a cross-reactive epitope in the hepatitis C virus nonstructural RNA polymerase–like protein. *J Virol* 66:4098–4106.

18. Rehermann B, K-M Chang, J McHutchinson, R Kokka, M Houghton, CM Rice, F Chisari. 1996. Differential cytotoxic T-lymphocyte responsiveness to hepatitis B and C viruses in chronically infected patients. *J Virol* 70:7092–7102.

19. Botarelli P, MR Brunetto, MA Minutello, P Calvo, D Unutmaz, AJ Weiner, QL Choo, JR Shuster, G Kuo, F Bonino, M Houghton, S Abrignani. 1993. T-lymphocyte response to hepatitis C virus in different clinical courses of infection. *Gastroenterology* 104:580–587.

20. Bakir TMF, M Halawani, MN Al-Ahdal, G Kessie, S Ramia. 1997. Significance of serum hepatitis C virus RNA, IgM and IgG antibodies as markers of hepatitis C infection. *Med Sci Res* 25:853–854.

21. Bui LA, LH Butterfield, JY Kim, A Ribas, P Seu, R Lau, JA Glaspy, WH McBride, JS Economou. 1997. In vivo therapy of hepatocellular carcinoma with a tumor-specific adenoviral vector expressing interleukin-2. *Hum Gene Ther* 8:2173–2182.

22. Seeff LB. 1997. Natural history of hepatitis C. *Hepatology* 26(suppl. 1): 21S–28S.

23. Di Bisceglie AM. 1997. Hepatitis C and hepatocellular carcinoma. *Hepatology* 26(suppl. 1):34S–38S.

24. Gretch DR. 1997. Diagnostic tests for hepatitis C. *Hepatology* 26(suppl. 1):43S–47S.

25. Lok ASF, NT Gunaratnam. 1997. Diagnosis of hepatitis C. *Hepatology* 26 (suppl. 1):48S–56S.
26. Perrillo RP. 1997. The role of liver biopsy in hepatitis C. *Hepatology* 26 (suppl. 1):57S–61S.
27. Alter MJ. 1997. Epidemiology of hepatitis C. *Hepatology* 26(suppl. 1): 62S–65S.
28. Merz M, M Seiberling, G Höxter, ML Hölting, HP Wortha. 1997. Elevation of liver enzymes in multiple dose trials during placebo treatment: are they predictable? *J Clin Pharmacol* 37:791–798.
29. Smith DB, P Simmonds. 1997. Characteristics of nucleotide substitution in the hepatitis C virus genome: constraints on sequence change in coding regions at both ends of the genome. *J Mol Evol* 45:238–246.
30. Tsai JF, JE Jeng, MS Ho, WY Chang, MY Hsieh, ZY Lin, JH Tsai. 1997. Effect of hepatitis C and B virus infection on risk of hepatocellular carcinoma: a prospective study. *Br J Cancer* 76:968–974.
31. McHugh TM, MK Viele, ES Chase, DJ Recktenwald. 1997. The sensitive detection and quantitation of antibody to hepatitis C by using a microsphere-based immunoassay and flow cytometry. *Cytometry* 29:106–112.
32. Nagy H, Y Panis, M Fabre, H Perrin, D Klatzmann, D Houssin. 1998. Are hepatomas a good target for suicide gene therapy? An experimental study in rats using retroviral-mediated transfer of thymidine kinase gene. *Surgery* 123:19–24.
33. Osna N, G Silonova, N Vilgert, E Hagina, V Kuse, V Giedraitis, A Zvirbliene, M Mauricas, A Sochnev. 1997. Chronic hepatitis C: T-helper1/T-helper2 imbalance could cause virus persistence in peripheral blood. *Scand J Clin Lab Invest* 57:703–710.
34. Farci P, J Bukh, RH Purcell. 1997. The quasispecies of hepatitis C virus and the host immune response. *Springer Semin Immunopathol* 19:5–26.
35. Abrignani S. 1997. Immune responses throughout hepatitis C virus (HCV) infection: hepatitis C from the immune system point of view. *Springer Semin Immunopathol* 19:47–55.
36. Chang KM, B Rehermann, FV Chisari. 1997. Immunopathology of hepatitis C. *Springer Semin Immunopathol* 19:57–68.
37. Koziel MJ, BD Walker. 1997. Characteristics of the intrahepatic cytotoxic T lymphocyte response in chronic hepatitis C virus infection. *Springer Semin Immunopathol* 19:69–83.
38. Walker CM. 1997. Comparative features of hepatitis C virus infection in humans and chimpanzees. *Springer Semin Immunopathol* 19:85–98.
39. Nolandt O, V Kern, H Müller, E Pfaff, L Theilmann, R Welker, HG Kräusslich. 1997. Analysis of hepatitis C virus core protein interaction domains. *J Gen Virol* 78:1331–1340.
40. Papatheodoridis GV, JK Delladetsima, A Katsoulidou, V Sypsa, M Albrecht, G Michel, A Hatzakis, NC Tassopoulos. 1997. Significance of IgM anti-hepatitis C core level in chronic hepatitis C. *J Hepatol* 27:36–41.
41. Pawlotsky JM, I Lonjon, C Hezode, B Raynard, F Darthuy, J Remire, CJ Soussy, D Dhumeaux. 1998. What strategy should be used for diagnosis

of hepatitis C virus infection in clinical laboratories? *Hepatology* 27: 1700–1702.

Chapters 4, Hepatitis C and End-Stage Liver Disease; 5, Hepatitis C and Liver Transplantation

1. Abbasoglu O, MF Levy, BB Brkic, G Testa, DR Jeyarajah, RM Goldstein, BS Husberg, TA Gonwa, GB Klintmalm. 1997. Ten years of liver transplantation—an evolving understanding of late graft loss. *Transplantation* 64:1801–1807.
2. Smith, BC, J Grove, MA Guzail, CP Day, AK Daly, AD Burt, MF Bassendine. 1998. Heterozygosity for hereditary hemochromatosis is associated with more fibrosis in chronic hepatitis C. *Hepatology* 27:1695–1699.
3. Tisone G, L Baiocchi, G Orlando, C Gandin, J Romagnoli, M Cepparulo, F Pisani, M Angelico, CU Casciani. 1998. Liver transplantation for hepatitis C virus end-stage liver cirrhosis as compared with other nonviral indications. *Transplant Proc* 30:696–697.
4. Poynard T, P Bedossa, P Opolon. 1997. Natural history of liver fibrosis progression in patients with chronic hepatitis C. *Lancet* 349:825–832.
5. Sheiner PA, P Boros, FM Klion, SN Thung, LK Schluger, JY Lau, E Mor, C Bodian, SR Guy, ME Schwartz, S Emre, HC Bodenheimer Jr, CM Miller. 1998. The efficacy of prophylactic interferon alfa-2b in preventing recurrent hepatitis C after liver transplantation. *Hepatology* 28(3): 831–838.
6. Otto G, GM Richter, L Theilmann, J Arnold, N Senninger, WJ Hofmann, C Herfarth. 1992. Liver transplantation after trans-jugular intrahepatic portosystemic stent shunt. *Chirurg* 63(9):730–732.
7. Carey WD. 1989. Evaluating treatment options for chronic liver disease. *Clevel Clin J Med* 56(5):473–474.
8. Gentilini P, G Laffi, G La Villa, RG Romanelli, G Buzzelli, V Casini-Raggi, L Melani, R Mazzanti, D Riccardi, M Pinzani, AL Zignego. 1997. Long course and prognostic factors of virus-induced cirrhosis of the liver. *Am J Gastroenterol* 92(1):66–72.
9. Knobler H, A Stagnaro-Green, S Wallenstein, M Schwartz, SH Roman. 1998. Higher incidence of diabetes in liver transplant recipients with hepatitis C. *J Clin Gastroenterol* 26(1):30–33.
10. Gane EJ, BC Portmann, NV Naoumov, HM Smith, JA Underhill, PT Donaldson, G Maertens, R Williams. 1996. Long-term outcome of hepatitis C infection after liver transplantation. *N Engl J Med* 334(13): 815–820.
11. Pol S, V Garrigue, C Legendre. 1996. Long-term outcome of hepatitis C infection after liver transplantation. *N Engl J Med* 335(7):522; discussion 522–523.

12. Fishman JA, RH Rubin, MJ Koziel, BJ Periera. 1996. Hepatitis C virus and organ transplantation. *Transplantation* 62(2):147–154.
13. Kizilisik TA, M al-Sebayel, A Hammad, I al-Traif, CG Ramirez, A Abdulla. 1997. Hepatitis C recurrence in liver transplant recipients. *Transplant Proc* 29(7):2875–2877.
14. Bouthot BA, BV Murthy, CH Schmid, AS Levey, BJ Pereira. 1997. Long-term follow-up of hepatitis C virus infection among organ transplant recipients: implications for policies on organ procurement. *Transplantation* 63(6):849–853.
15. National Institutes of Health. 1997. Consensus development conference panel statement: management of hepatitis C. *Hepatology* 26(3)(suppl. 1): 2S–10S.

Chapter 6, Stopping the Spread of Hepatitis C: Blood Transfusions, Recreational Drug Use, Sex, Tattoos, Acupuncture, Manicures, Pedicures, and Body Piercing

1. National Institutes of Health. 1997. Consensus development conference panel statement: management of hepatitis C. *Hepatology* 26(3)(suppl. 1): 2S–10S.
2. Karmochkine, M, F Carrat, AJ Valleron, G Raguin. 1998. Modes of hepatitis C virus transmission. *Presse Med* 27:871–876.
3. Shiffman ML. 1998. Management of hepatitis C. DDW prototype. *Clin Perspect Gastroenterol* 6–19.
4. Bronowicki JP, V Venard, C Botté, N Monhoven, I Gastin, L Choné, H Hudziak, B Rhin, C Delanoæ, A LeFaou, MA Bigard, P Gaucher. 1997. Patient-to-patient transmission of hepatitis C virus during colonoscopy. *N Engl J Med* 337:237–240.
5. Alter MJ. 1993. The detection, transmission, and outcome of hepatitis C infection. *Infect Agents Dis* 2:155–166.
6. Heintges T, JR Wands. 1997. Hepatitis C virus: epidemiology and transmission. *Hepatology* 26:521–526.
7. Hoofnagle JH, TS Tralka. 1997. The National Institutes of Health consensus development conference: management of hepatitis C—introduction. *Hepatology* 26(suppl. 1):1S.
8. Alter HJ, C Conry-Cantilena, J Melpolder, D Tan, M Van Raden, D Herion, D Lau, JH Hoofnagle. 1997. Hepatitis C in asymptomatic blood donors. *Hepatology* 26(suppl. 1):29S–33S.
9. Alter, MJ. 1997. Epidemiology of hepatitis C. *Hepatology* 26(suppl. 1): 62S–65S.
10. Dienstag JL. 1997. Sexual and perinatal transmission of hepatitis C. *Hepatology* 26(suppl. 1):66S–70S.

11. Gitlin N, FS Nolte, M Weiss. 1997. Hepatitis C: risk of a haircut. *Ann Intern Med* 126:410–411.
12. Brambilla A, R Pristera, F Salvatori, G Poli, E Vicenzi. 1997. Transmission of HIV-1 and hepatitis C by head-butting. *Lancet* 350:1370.
13. Kozarek RA. 1997. Transmission of hepatitis C virus during colonoscopy. *N Engl J Med* 337:1848–1849.
14. Van der Poel CL, F Ebeling. 1998. Hepatitis C virus: epidemiology, transmission and prevention. *Curr Stud Hematol Blood Transfus* 62:208–236.

Chapter 7, Hepatitis C and Alcohol

1. National Institutes of Health. 1997. Consensus development conference panel statement: management of hepatitis C. *Hepatology* 26(3)(suppl. 1): 2S–10S.
2. Schiff ER. 1997. Hepatitis C and alcohol. *Hepatology* 26(suppl. 1):39S–42S.
3. Corrao G, S Aricò. 1998. Independent and combined action of hepatitis C virus infection and alcohol consumption on the risk of symptomatic liver cirrhosis. *Hepatology* 27:914–919.
4. Stroffolini T. 1998. Alcohol, hepatitis C infection, and liver cirrhosis: is the cup half full or half empty? *J Hepatol* 28:728–730.
5. Seeff LB. 1997. Chronic hepatitis C: Beware the older drinking male: fibrosis progression beckons! Comments. *Hepatology* 26:1074–1076.
6. Sachithanandan S, E Kay, M Leader, JF Fielding. 1997. The effect of light drinking on hepatitis C liver disease: the jury is still out. *Biomed Pharmacother* 51:295–297.
7. Ostapowicz G, KJR Watson, SA Locarnini, PV Desmond. 1998. Role of alcohol in the progression of liver disease caused by hepatitis C virus infection. *Hepatology* 27:1730–1735.
8. Diehl AM. 1998. Effects of chronic ethanol consumption on cytokine regulation of liver regeneration. *Alcohol Clin Exp Res* 22:762–763.

Chapter 8, The Search for the Holy Grail

1. Moriya K, H Yotsuyanagi, Y Shintani, H Fujie, K Ishibashi, Y Matsuura, T Miyamura, K Koike. 1997. Hepatitis C virus core protein induces hepatic steatosis in transgenic mice. *J Gen Virol* 78:1527–1531.
2. Siriboonkoom W, Gramlich L. 1998. Nutrition and chronic liver disease. *Can J Gastroenterol* 12(3):201–207.
3. Chin SE, RW Shepherd, BJ Thomas, GJ Cleghorn, MK Patrick, JA Wilcox, TH Ong, SV Lynch, R Strong. 1992. Nutritional support in chil-

dren with end-stage liver disease: a randomized crossover trial of a branched-chain amino acid supplement. *Am J Clin Nutr* 56(1):158–163.
4. Simko V. 1985. Nutrition therapy for liver disease. *Comprehens Ther* 11(12):62–67.
5. Novy MA, KB Schwarz. 1997. Nutritional considerations and management of the child with liver disease. *Nutrition* 13(3):177–184.
6. Corish C. 1997. Nutrition and liver disease. *Nutr Rev* 55(1 Pt 1):17–20.

Chapters 9, Diet and Nutrition; 10, Hepatitis C and Interferon

1. National Institutes of Health. 1997. Consensus development conference panel statement: management of hepatitis C. *Hepatology* 26(3)(suppl. 1): 2S–10S.
2. Shiffman ML, CM Hofmann, EB Thompson, A Ferreira-Gonzalez, MJ Contos, A Koshy, VA Luketic, AJ Sanyal, AS Mills, C Garrett. 1997. Relationship between biochemical, virologic and histologic response during interferon treatment of chronic hepatitis C. *Hepatology* 26: 780–785.
3. Ohkawa K, N Yuki, Y Kanazawa, K Ueda, E Mita, Y Sasaki, A Kasahara, N Hayashi. 1997. Cleavage of viral RNA and inhibition of viral translation by hepatitis C virus RNA-specific hammerhead ribozyme in vitro. *J Hepatol* 27:78–84.
4. Mamounas M, M Yu. 1996. Applications of gene therapy for HIV and hepatitis B and C virus infections. *Infect Med* 13:817–823.
5. Polyak SJ, G Faulkner, RL Carithers Jr, L Corey, DR Gretch. 1997. Assessment of hepatitis C virus quasispecies heterogeneity by gel shift analysis: correlation with response to interferon therapy. *J Infect Dis* 175:1101–1107.
6. Lindsay KL 1997. Therapy of hepatitis C: overview. *Hepatology* 26(suppl. 1):71S–77S.
7. Carithers RL Jr, SS Emerson. 1997. Therapy of hepatitis C: meta-analysis of interferon alfa-2b trials. *Hepatology* 26(suppl. 1):83S–88S.
8. Di Stefano G, FP Colonna, A Bongini, C Busi, A Mattioli, L Fiume. 1997. Ribavirin conjugated with lactosaminated poly-L-lysine—selective delivery to the liver and increased antiviral activity in mice with viral hepatitis. *Biochem Pharmacol* 54:357–363.
9. Shiffman ML. 1998. Management of hepatitis C. DDW prototype. *Clin Perspect Gastroenterol* 6–19.
10. Urvil PT, N Kakiuchi, DM Zhou, K Shimotohno, PKR Kumar, S Nishikawa. 1997. Selection of RNA aptamers that bind specifically to the NS3 protease of hepatitis C virus. *Eur J Biochem* 248:130–138.
11. Lee WM. 1997. Therapy of hepatitis C: interferon alfa-2a trials. *Hepatology* 26(suppl. 1):89S–95S.

12. Farrell GC. 1997. Therapy of hepatitis C: interferon alfa-nl trials. *Hepatology* 26(suppl. 1):96S–100S.
13. Keeffe, EB, FB Hollinger, R Bailey, VG Bain, K Bala, L Balart, M Black, H Bonkovsky, W Cassidy, JR Craig, J Donovan, GM Dusheiko, M Ehrinpreis, G Everson, S Feinman, RT Foust, H Fromm, S Hauser, EJ Heathcote, JC Hoefs, E Hunter, S James, DM Jensen, P Killenberg. 1997. Therapy of hepatitis C: consensus interferon trials. *Hepatology* 26(suppl. 1):101S–107S.
14. Reichard O, R Schvarcz, O Weiland. 1997. Therapy of hepatitis C: alpha interferon and ribavirin. *Hepatology* 26(suppl. 1):108S–111S.
15. Dusheiko G. 1997. Side effects of alpha interferon in chronic hepatitis C. *Hepatology* 26(suppl. 1):112S–121S.
16. Davis GL, JYN Lau. 1997. Factors predictive of a beneficial response to therapy of hepatitis C. *Hepatology* 26(suppl. 1):122S–127S.
17. Schalm SW, G Fattovich, JT Brouwer. 1997. Therapy of hepatitis C: patients with cirrhosis. *Hepatology* 26(suppl. 1):128S–132S.
18. Marcellin P, S Levy, S Erlinger. 1997. Therapy of hepatitis C: patients with normal aminotransferase levels. *Hepatology* 26(suppl. 1):133S–136S.
19. Alberti A, L Chemello, F Noventa, L Cavalletto, G De Salvo. 1997. Therapy of hepatitis C: re-treatment with alpha interferon. *Hepatology* 26 (suppl. 1):137S–142S.
20. Bonkovsky HL 1997. Therapy of hepatitis C: other options. *Hepatology* 26(suppl. 1):143S–151S.
21. Von Weizsäcker F, S Wieland, J Köck, WB Offensperger, S Offensperger, D Moradpour, HE Blum. 1997. Gene therapy for chronic viral hepatitis: ribozymes, antisense oligonucleotides, and dominant negative mutants. *Hepatology* 26:251–255.
22. Liu MA. 1997. The immunologist's grail: vaccines that generate cellular immunity. *Proc Natl Acad Sci USA* 94:10496–10498.
23. Rondon IJ, WA Marasco. 1997. Intracellular antibodies (intrabodies) for gene therapy of infectious diseases. *Annu Rev Microbiol* 51:257–283.
24. Marcellin P, N Boyer, A Gervais, M Martinot, M Pouteau, C Caselnau, A Kilani, J Areias, A Auperin, JP Benhamou, C Degott, S Erlinger. 1997. Long term improvement and loss of detectable intrahepatic HCV-RNA in patients with chronic hepatitis C and sustained respone to interferon alpha-therapy. *Ann Intern Med* 127:875–881.
25. Gavier B, MA Martínez-González, JI Riezu-Boj, JJ Lasarte, N Garcia, MP Civeira, J Prieto. 1997. Viremia after one month of interferon therapy predicts treatment outcome in patients with chronic hepatitis C. *Gastroenterology* 113:1647–1653.
26. Farci P, J Bukh, RH Purcell. 1997. The quasispecies of hepatitis C virus and the host immune response. *Springer Semin Immunopathol* 19:5–26.
27. Imada K, Y Fukuda, Y Koyama, I Nakano, M Yamada, Y Katano, T Hayakawa. 1997. Naive and memory T cell infiltrates in chronic hepatitis C: phenotypic changes with interferon treatment. *Clin Exp Immunol* 109: 59–66.

28. Lemon SM. 1997. Targeting the Achilles' heel of hepatitis C virus. *Hepatology* 25:1035–1037.
29. Alt M, R Renz, PH Hofschneider, WH Caselmann. 1997. Core specific antisense phosphorothioate oligodeoxynucleotides as potent and specific inhibitors of hepatitis C viral translation. *Arch Virol* 142:589–599.
30. Yasui K, T Okanoue, Y Murakami, Y Itoh, M Minami, S Sakamoto, M Sakamoto, K Nishioji. 1998. Dynamics of hepatitis C viremia following interferon-α administration. *J Infect Dis* 177:1475–1479.
31. Hoofnagle, JH, KD Mullen, DB Jones, et al. 1986. Treatment of chronic non-A non-B hepatitis with recombinant human alpha interferon: a preliminary report. *N Engl J Med* 315:1575–1578.
32. Lau, DT-Y, DE Kleiner, MG Ghany, Y Park, P Schmid, JH Hoofnagle. 1998. 10-Year follow-up after interferon-alpha therapy for chronic hepatitis C. *Hepatology* 28(4):1121–1127.

Chapter 11, Alternative Medicine or Unconventional Medicine

1. Von Herbay A, W Stahl, C Niederau, H Sies. 1997. Vitamin E improves the aminotransferase status of patients suffering from viral hepatitis C: a randomized, double-blind, placebo-controlled study. *Free Radic Res* 27: 599–605.
2. Parés A, R Planas, M Torres, J Caballería, JM Viver, D Acero, J Panés, J Rigau, J Santos, J Rodés. 1998. Effects of silymarin in alcoholic patients with cirrhosis of the liver: results of a controlled, double-blind, randomized and multicenter trial. *J Hepatol* 28:615–621.
3. Merz M, M Seiberling, G Höxter, ML Hölting, HP Wortha. 1997. Elevation of liver enzymes in multiple dose trials during placebo treatment: are they predictable? *J Clin Pharmacol* 37:791–798.
4. Wolf GM, LM Petrovic, SE Roijter, et al. 1994. Acute hepatitis associated with the Chinese herbal product jin bu huan. *Ann Intern Med* 1212:729–735.
5. Itoh S, K Marutani, T Nishijima, et al. 1995. Liver injuries induced by herbal medicine, syosaiko-to. *Dig Dis Sci* 40:1845–1848.
6. Bach N, SN Thung, F Schaffner. 1989. Comfrey herb tea–induced hepatic veno-occlusive disease. *Am J Med* 87:97–99.
7. Anonymous. 1998. When patients want alternative care. *ACP-ASIM Observer* 18(7):1, 20.

Chapter 12, The Body's Efforts to Fight Hepatitis C, and Potential Vaccines

1. Koziel MJ, D Dudley, N Afdhal, A Grakoui, CM Rice, QL Choo, M Houghton, BD Walker. 1995. HLA class I-restricted cytotoxic T lympho-

cytes specific for hepatitis C virus: identification of multiple epitopes and characterization of patterns of cytokine release. *J Clin Invest* 96:2311–2321.

2. Hitomi Y, WM McDonnell, F Askari. 1994. Hepatitis C core protein as a possible vaccine against Hepatitis C. *Hepatology* 20(4,2):230A.

3. Ulmer JB, JJ Donnelly, SE Parker, GH Rhodes, PL Felgner, MA Liu. 1993. Heterologous protection against influenza by injection of DNA encoding a viral protein. *Science* 259:1745–1749.

4. Askari FK, H Li, S Dasgupta, WM McDonnell. 1997. Immunostimulatory elements (ISS) augment the immune response to hepatitis C core protein plasmid expression vectors: a step toward an improved vaccine for hepatitis C. *Hepatology* 26(4,2):407A.

5. Choo QL, G Kuo, R Ralston, et al. 1994. Vaccination of chimpanzees against infection by the hepatitis C virus. *Proc Natl Acad Sci USA* 91: 1294–1298.

6. Farci P, HJ Alter, DC Wong, RH Miller, S Govindarajan, R Engle, M Shapiro, RH Purcell. 1994. Prevention of hepatitis C virus infection in chimpanzees after antibody-mediated in vitro neutralization. *Proc Natl Acad Sci USA* 91:7792–7796.

7. Hitomi Y, WM McDonnell, J Baker, FK Askari. 1995. Analysis of the prokaryotic expression of the hepatitis C core protein and the murine immune response to recombinant protein. *Viral Immunol* 8(2):109–119.

8. Martin LP, L Lau, M Asano, R Ahmed. 1995. DNA vaccination against persistent viral infection. *J Virol* 69:2574–2582.

9. McDonnell WM. 1993. Gene transfer as a new mode of vaccination: implications for hepatitis C. *Hepatol* 18:694–698.

10. Hitomi Y, WM McDonnell, AA Killeen, FK Askari. 1995. Sequence analysis of the hepatitis C virus core gene suggests the core protein as an appropriate target for hepatitis C vaccine strategies. *J Viral Hepatitis* 2(5):235–241.

11. Klinman DM, G Yamshchikov, Y Ishigatsubo. 1997. Contribution of CpG motifs to the immunogenicity of DNA vaccines. *J Immunol* 158:3635–3639.

12. Sato Y, M Roman, H Tighe, D Lee, M Corr, MD Nguyen, GJ Silverman, M Lotz, DA Carson, E Raz. 1996. Immunostimulatory DNA sequences necessary for effective intradermal gene immunization. *Science* 273: 352–354.

13. Donnelly JJ, A Friedman, D Martinez, DL Montgomery, JW Shiver, SL Motzel, JB Ulmer, MA Liu. 1995. Preclinical efficacy of a prototype DNA vaccine: enhanced protection against antigenic drift in influenza virus. *Nature Med* 1:583–587.

14. Major ME, L Vitvitski, MA Mink, M Schleef, RG Whalen, C Trepo, G Inchauspe. 1995. DNA-based immunization with chimeric vectors for the induction of immune responses against the hepatitis C virus nucleocapsid. *J Virol* 69:5798–5805.

15. Saito, T, GJ Sherman, K Kurokohchi, ZP Guo, M Donets, MYW Yu, JA Berzofsky, T Akatsuka, SM Feinstone. 1997. Plasmid DNA-based immunization for hepatitis C virus structural proteins: immune responses in mice. *Gastroenterology* 112:1321–1330.
16. Koziel MJ, TJ Liang. 1997. DNA vaccines and viral hepatitis: are we going around in circles? *Gastroenterology* 112:1410–1414.
17. Kawamura T, A Furusaka, MJ Koziel, RT Chung, TC Wang, EV Schmidt, TJ Liang. 1997. Transgenic expression of hepatitis C virus structural proteins in the mouse. *Hepatology* 25:1014–1021.
18. McDonnell WM, FK Askari. 1996. Molecular Medicine: DNA vaccines. *N Engl J Med* 334(1):42–45.
19. Lagging LM, K Meyer, D Hoft, M Houghton, RB Belshe, R Ray. 1995. Immune response to plasmid DNA encoding the hepatitis C virus core protein. *J Virol* 69:5859–5863.
20. Tokushige K, T Wakita, C Pachuk, D Moradpour, DB Weiner, VR Zurawski, JR Wands. 1996. Expression and immune response to hepatitis C virus core DNA-based vaccine constructs. *Hepatology* 1:14–20.
21. Saito T, GJ Sherman, K Kurokohchi, Z-P Guo, M Donets, M-YM Yu, JA Berzofsky, T Akatsuka, SM Feinstone. 1997. Plasmid DNA-based immunization for hepatitis C virus structural proteins: immune responses in mice. *Gastroenterology* 112:1321–1330.
22. Wilson JM, FK Askari. 1996. Hepatic and gastrointestinal gene therapy. In: Yamada T, ed. *Textbook of Gastroenterology: Gastroenterology Updates*. Philadelphia: J.B. Lippincott Co., Vol. 1(5):1–20.
23. Tang DC, M DeVit, SA Johnston. 1992. Genetic immunization is a simple method for elicitng an immune response. *Nature* 356:152–154.
24. Garcon NM, HR Six. 1991. Universal vaccine carrier. Liposomes that provide T-dependent help to weak antigens. *J Immunol* 146:3697–3702.
25. Anonymous. 1997. Vaccines at risk. *Nature* 389:647.
26. Chattergoon M, J Boyer, DB Weiner. 1997. Genetic immunization: a new era in vaccines and immune therapeutics. *FASEB J* 11:753–763.
27. Pieroni L, E Santolini, C Fipaldini, L Pacini, G Migliaccio, N La Monica. 1997. In vitro study of the NS2-3 protease of hepatitis C virus. *J Virol* 71: 6373–6380.
28. Chen CM, LR You, LH Hwang, YHW Lee. 1997. Direct interaction of hepatitis C virus core protein with the cellular lymphotoxin-b receptor modulates the signal pathway of the lymphotoxin-b receptor. *J Virol* 71: 9417–9426.
29. Inchauspé G. 1997. Gene vaccination for hepatitis C. *Springer Semin Immunopathol* 19:211–221.
30. McDonnell WM, FK Askari. 1997. Immunization. *JAMA* 278:2000–2007.
31. Triyatni M., AR Jilbert, M Qiao, DS Miller, CJ Burrell. 1998. Protective efficacy of DNA vaccines against duck hepatitis B virus infection. *J Virol* 72:84–94.
32. Muramatsu S, S Ishido, T Fujita, M Itoh, H Hotta. 1997. Nuclear localiza-

tion of the NS3 protein of hepatitis C virus and factors affecting the localization. *J Virol* 71:4954–4961.

33. Cribier B, C Schmitt, D Rey, JM Lang, A Kirn, F Stoll-Keller. 1998. Production of cytokines in patients infected by hepatitis C virus. *J Med Virol* 55:89–91.

Chapters 13, Your Skin and Joints: Effects of Hepatitis C Outside the Liver; 14, Hepatitis C and Your Kidneys; 15, Your Immune System

1. Bonkovsky HL, M Poh-Fitzpatrick, N Pimstone, J Obando, A Di Bisceglie, C Tattrie, K Tortorelli, P LeClair, MG Mercurio, RW Lambrecht. 1998. Porphyria cutanea tarda, hepatitis C, and HFE gene mutations in North America. *Hepatology* 27:1661–1669.
2. Barkhuizen A, RM Bennett. 1997. Hepatitis C infection presenting with rheumatic manifestations. *J Rheumatol* 24:1238.
3. Durand JM. 1997. Extrahepatic manifestations of hepatitis C virus manifestations positively-related to hepatitis C virus. *Presse Med* 26:1014–1022.
4. Cimmino MA, A Picciotto, N Sinelli, R Brizzolara, S Accardo. 1997. Has hepatitis C virus a specific tropism for the synovial membrane? *Br J Rheumatol* 36:505–506.
5. Hassoun AAK, TB Nippoldt, RD Tiegs, S Khosla. 1997. Hepatitis C-associated osteosclerosis: An unusual syndrome of acquired osteosclerosis in adults. *Am J Med* 103:70–73.
6. Buskila D, A Shnaider, L Neumann, D Zilberman, N Hilzenrat, E Sikuler. 1997. Fibromyalgia in hepatitis C virus infection—another infectious disease relationship. *Arch Intern Med* 157:2497–2500.
7. O'Connor WJ, G Murphy, C Darby, F Mulcahy, R O'Moore, L Barnes. 1997. Type of impaired porphyrin metabolism caused by hepatitis C virus is not porphyria cutanea tarda but chronic hepatic porphyria. Reply. *Arch Dermatol* 133:1171.
8. Shaker JL, WR Reinus, MP Whyte. 1998. Hepatitis C-associated osteosclerosis: late onset after blood transfusion in an elderly woman. *J Clin Endocrinol Metab* 83:93–98.
9. Akriviadis EA, I Xanthakis, C Navrozidou, A Papadopoulos. 1997. Prevalence of cryoglobulinemia in chronic hepatitis C virus infection and response to treatment with interferon-alpha. *J Clin Gastroenterol* 25(4): 612–618.
10. Hadziyannis SJ. 1997. The spectrum of extrahepatic manifestations in hepatitis C virus infection. *J Viral Hepatitis* 4(1):9–28.
11. Gordon SC. 1996. Extrahepatic manifestations of hepatitis C. *Dig Dis* 14(3):157–168.

12. Stehman-Breen C, CE Alpers, WG Couser, R Willson, RJ Johnson. 1995. Hepatitis C virus associated membranous glomerulonephritis. *Clin Nephrol* 44(3):141–147.
13. Parke AL, DV Parke. 1994. Hepatic disease, the gastrointestinal tract, and rheumatic disease. *Curr Opin Rheumatol* 6(1):85–94.
14. Sham RL, CY Ou, J Cappuccio, C Braggins, K Dunnigan, PD Phatak. 1997. Correlation between genotype and phenotype in hereditary hemochromatosis: analysis of 61 cases. *Blood Cells Mol Dis* 23:314–320.
15. Gomi H, K Hatanaka, T Miura, I Matsuo. 1997. Type of impaired porphyrin metabolism caused by hepatitis C virus is not porphyria cutanea tarda but chronic hepatic porphyria. *Arch Dermatol* 133:1170–1171.

Chapter 16, Psychological Impact of Hepatitis C

1. Hunt CM, JA Dominitz, BP Bute, B Waters, U Blasi, DM Williams. 1997. Effect of interferon-a treatment of chronic hepatitis C on health-related quality of life. *Dig Dis Sci* 42:2482–2486.
2. Foster GR, RD Goldin, HC Thomas. 1998. Chronic hepatitis C virus infection causes a significant reduction in quality of life in the absence of cirrhosis. *Hepatology* 27:209–212.
3. Bennett, WG, Y Inoue, JR Beck, JB Wong, SG Pauker, GL Davis. 1997. Estimates of the cost-effectiveness of a single course of interferon-a2b in patients with histologically mild chronic hepatitis C. *Ann Intern Med* 127:855–865.
4. Kim WR, JJ Poterucha, JE Hermans, TM Therneau, ER Dickson, RW Evans, JB Gross Jr. 1997. Cost-effectiveness of 6 and 12 months of interferon-a therapy for chronic hepatitis C. *Ann Intern Med* 127:866–874.
5. Koff RS. 1997. Therapy of hepatitis C: cost-effectiveness analysis. *Hepatology* 26(suppl. 1):152S–155S.

Chapter 17, Epilogue

1. National Institutes of Health. 1997. Consensus development conference panel statement: management of hepatitis C. *Hepatology* 26(3)(suppl. 1):2S–10S.
2. Everhart JE, M Stolar, JH Hoofnagle. 1997. Management of hepatitis C: a national survey of gastroenterologists and hepatologists. *Hepatology* 26(suppl. 1):78S–82S.
3. Shiffman ML. 1998. Management of hepatitis C. DDW prototype. *Clin Perspect Gastroenterol* 6–19.

Glossary

One of the reasons it can be difficult to communicate with doctors is that they use a different vocabulary from nonmedical people. Here is a brief glossary of liver disease terms which may serve to clarify terms the patient and his family may encounter. **CAUTION: List of drug side effects and uses is not meant to be complete. Consult a physician, pharmacist or appropriate reference for more detailed and complete information.**

Abdomen—the area of the body below the rib cage and above the legs, which contains the stomach, liver, spleen, and bowels. On the surface of the body the abdomen's defining feature is the umbilicus, or belly button.

Acute hepatitis—inflammation in the liver of fewer than 6 months' duration. Common causes include viral hepatitis, drug reactions, autoimmune hepatitis, and Wilson's disease, a disorder of copper metabolism which leads to accumulation of copper in the liver, resulting in liver fibrosis.

Albumin—a protein or molecule made in the liver which circulates in high concentration in the blood. Albumin functions to bind other molecules and drugs in the circulation, and also serves a significant function in holding fluid inside blood vessels. As serum albumin levels fall, fluid may seep out of blood vessels into the abdomen, leading to ascites (fluid accumulation in the abdomen) or ankle edema (fluid accumulation in the ankles). The serum albumin level is used as a long-term measure of liver synthetic function.

Aldactone—a diuretic which promotes urination and retention of potassium. A very useful drug often prescribed in combination with furosemide, another type of diuretic, in the treatment of ascites. Side effects include increased serum potassium levels and breast tenderness.

Alpha-1 antitrypsin deficiency—a genetic disease that affects multiple organs including the liver in 20% of cases. The disease is characterized by the production of defective alpha-1 antitrypsin molecules in the liver which are improperly exported from liver cells. The accumulation of misfolded alpha-1 antitrypsin molecules in the liver can lead to liver damage and ultimately cirrhosis. The main hallmark of this disease is lung problems, as alpha-1 antitrypsin normally functions to protect the lungs from damage.

ALT—(a.k.a. SGPT) a liver enzyme which is measured in blood. Elevations in this blood value are consistent with hepatitis or inflammation of the liver. Often followed as a marker for response to treatment during a course of therapy for hepatitis C.

Antibody—a protein made by the immune system that recognizes and binds to a foreign invader or antigen to try to destroy it. Antibodies can be made to fight specific foreign antigens, and their identification in the blood may serve as a marker of prior or ongoing infection. Many diagnostic tests for hepatitis C infection look for antibodies to the hepatitis C virus.

Ascites—the accumulation of fluid within the abdomen. The presence of ascites is one of the hallmark features of hepatic decompensation. Ascites is often treated with di-uretics or paracentesis.

AST—(a.k.a. SGOT) a liver enzyme which is measured in blood. Elevations in this blood value are consistent with hepatitis or inflammation of the liver. Often followed as a marker for response to treatment during a course of therapy for hepatitis C.

Autoimmune hepatitis—a form of liver disease in which the body's own immune system attacks the liver, which leads to the immune system's injuring the liver. This disease is diagnosed through liver biopsies and inferred from serum tests of ANA (antinuclear antibody), ASM or (antismooth muscle antibody), or LKM (anti-LKM, liver–kidney antibody). This disease often responds to steroid treatment.

Bilirubin—a breakdown product of hemoglobin, which functions to carry oxygen in blood cells. This is a waste product which is normally eliminated from the body through the liver. As bilirubin levels build up in the body, they give the skin and eyes a characteristic yellow color, called jaundice. Long-term marked elevations of bilirubin can lead to damage to nerve cells, but this is generally not a problem in patients with liver disease from hepatitis C.

Banding—a procedure used to treat or obliterate esophageal varices, which are bleeding-prone, thin-walled engorged blood vessels in the esophagus that can develop in end-stage liver disease. A small device that dispenses black rubber bands is attached to the end of the endoscope. The varices are then sucked up inside of the rubber band, and the band is next released around the engorged blood vessel. The band entraps this engorged vessel, causing tissue death and scarring of the area where the engorged blood vessel used to be. This can prevent variceal bleeding, which can be life-threatening.

Chronic hepatitis—generally defined as inflammation in the liver of greater than 6 months' duration. Causes include drugs, viruses, autoimmune liver disease, hemochromatosis

(iron overload) and Wilson's disease (copper overload).
Hepatitis C is the most common cause of chronic hepatitis.

Cirrhosis—the endpoint of many different kinds of liver disease. It involves extensive fibrosis or scarring over throughout the liver. Cirrhosis is generally felt to be irreversible. Cirrhosis can be broken down into two phases: stable cirrhosis, during which the liver continues to perform its normal functions, and unstable or decompensated cirrhosis, during which the liver is not able to keep up with all of its chores.

Consensus interferon, INFERGEN—a brand of interferon manufactured by the AMGEN pharmaceutical company. The structure or protein sequence of this interferon is intended to recapitulate a mixture of a number of slightly different interferon molecules in the hope it might have improved activity compared to other brands of interferon. To date, dramatic differences have not been shown.

Decompensated cirrhosis—also referred to as "unstable cirrhosis," decompensated cirrhosis consists of scarring over of the liver associated with symptoms of ascites (fluid accumulation in the abdomen), encephalopathy (confusion due to the buildup of toxins normally cleared by the liver in the body) or variceal bleeding (severe gastrointestinal bleeding caused by blood backing up through the liver). Liver transplantation should be considered at this time.

Diuretics—drugs that promote urination and allow the body to get rid of excess fluid and some salts. Often used to control ascites and accumulation of fluid in the lower extremities or edema.

Edema—accumulation of fluid in the soft tissues outside of blood vessels, particularly in the legs around the ankles. Severe edema can extend from the ankles and into the abdomen. One particularly frightening manifestation is when the scrotum becomes engorged with fluid in males.

Encephalopathy—hepatic encephalopathy is mental confusion caused by the buildup of toxic waste products in the body which the liver normally clears.

End-stage liver disease (ESLD)—the point of no return has been reached in cirrhosis, and decompensated or unstable cirrhosis has set in. At this time liver transplantation may be considered. Symptoms include muscle wasting, fatigue, ascites, encephalopathy, or variceal bleeding.

Essential mixed cryoglobulinemia—a complication of hepatitis C infection which occurs outside of the liver in 1–2% of infected individuals. Affected individuals have hepatitis C particles bound to antibodies circulating in their blood. When these particles deposit in small blood vessels in the hands, feet, or kidneys, they cause vascular inflammation or kidney injury (membranoproliferative glomerulonephritis).

Furosemide—a diuretic, a drug that makes you urinate. Promotes loss of sodium from the body, which can be beneficial for people with liver diseases, as they frequently have too much sodium in their bodies.

Hepatologist—physician who specializes in the treatment of individuals with liver disease. At least at one time, everyone with hepatitis C should be under this specialist's care.

Hemochromatosis—a disease of iron metabolism in which too much iron is absorbed through the gut and deposited in the liver, leading ultimately to cirrhosis. Other organs damaged by excess iron include the heart and kidneys. Skin may be darkened. Often inherited in an autosomal-recessive pattern. Genetic tests are available for the common mutations causing this disease. Treated by phlebotomy or bleeding treatments to reduce excess iron.

Hepatitis C (HCV)—a liver disease caused by the hepatitis C virus. The virus is transmitted through contaminated blood from other people who have the disease. The infection can be characterized by a prolonged symptomless period of chronic infection. Progresses to chronic hepatitis in the majority of infections, and may ultimately lead to cirrhosis, liver failure, and liver cancer. In technical terms, the virus is a positive stranded RNA virus of the Flaviviridae family. More directly, a microscopic infectious particle consisting of RNA which carries the instructions for making more viruses and several proteins, some of which cover the viral RNA molecule like an envelope conceals a letter.

Hepatitis C antibody—actually includes many different antibodies to a broad range of hepatitis C proteins. The initial test for antibodies usually is a straightforward EIA assay, in which plates are coated with hepatitis C proteins and blood that reacts with the hepatitis C proteins is developed to change color.

Hepatitis C RNA—a serum test performed to detect RNA derived from hepatitis C circulating in the bloodstream. Two tests are commonly employed—a qualitative test, which detects the presence or absence of hepatitis C RNA, and a generally less sensitive but more quantitative test which assigns a specific numerical value to the quantity of hepatitis C RNA circulating in the bloodstream. Initially viewed as an experimental test, hepatitis C RNA levels are being used more frequently to confirm active infection with the hepatitis C virus.

HIV—human immunodeficiency virus, the virus that causes AIDS. Many patients with HIV also are infected with hepatitis C.

INTRON A—a brand of interferon manufactured by the Schering-Plough Corporation.

Interferon—a naturally occurring class of proteins used to stimulate the immune system to fight hepatitis and certain forms of cancer. When used to fight hepatitis C, individual responses to treatment may be divided into three broad categories: (1) sustained responders who rid the virus from their blood and have their serum liver enzymes return to normal even 6 months after therapy is stopped; (2) nonresponders, who do not show a disappearance of viral RNA levels from the blood and do not have their serum liver enzymes return to normal; (3) partial responders, who drop their viral levels and liver enzymes on treatment but fail to maintain these successes once treatment is discontinued.

Jaundice—The characteristic yellow color seen in the skin and eyes as bilirubin levels build up in the body, usually from liver dysfunction or blockage of the bile ducts leading from the liver to the small bowel. May also be seen with hemolysis or excessive breakdown of blood cells.

Lactulose—a medicine given to treat hepatic encephalopathy or confusion resulting from the buildup of toxins normally eliminated from the body by the liver. Lactulose is a nonabsorbable fluid that promotes loose bowel movements, helping to eliminate the toxins from the body that are normally cleared by the liver. Taken as a liquid, the dose is generally increased or decreased to achieve two to four loose bowel movements per day.

Liver biopsy—a sample of liver tissue taken to be examined under a microscope. The "gold standard" in terms of defining the extent of liver disease and prognosis, the liver biopsy also often helps to determine the cause of the liver disease. The biopsy may be taken with a needle through the skin, through a catheter which passes through the blood vessels from the neck down into the liver, or at the time of open or laparoscopic surgery.

Liver function tests (LFTs)—these generally consist of the albumin, which is a long-term measure of liver synthetic function, the transaminases or liver enzymes, as defined below, and the total bilirubin level. Liver function tests are one marker of the severity of liver disease and can be a useful measure of ongoing liver injury. They may also be used to differentiate between injury to liver cells or hepatocytes and blockage of the biliary tree which drains bile from the liver to the small bowel.

Multidose pen—an applicator to make interferon treatment more convenient by providing the drug in a prefilled pen-like reservoir with dial-in-dosing control. The desired dose of interferon is selected and then injected under the skin using a needle attached to the barrel of the pen. Must be refrigerated between doses.

PCR—polymerase chain reaction. PCR is used to copy and amplify small quantities of RNA or DNA so that they can be detected. Using PCR tests specific for hepatitis C, it is possible to detect minuscule quantities of hepatitis C RNA by amplifying or copying these sequences over and over again. Now used in many routine diagnostic tests in medicine, PCR was initially used primarily as a research tool.

Paracentesis—the technique whereby a needle is inserted into the abdomen to tap excess fluid or ascites. When termed a diagnostic paracentesis, the purpose is to send some of the fluid to the laboratory to look for infection or cancer or help determine the reason for the ascites. When termed a therapeutic paracentesis, fluid is drained off to relieve liquid overload from the abdomen. The procedure is done with the patient awake, using local anesthesia at the site of needle insertion.

Prothrombin time (PT)—an excellent marker of short-term liver function, the prothrombin time is a measure of blood clotting. Since many of the proteins that help blood clot are manufactured in the liver, the prothrombin time increases as the liver fails. Since the clotting factors are constantly being made, degraded, and replenished, the prothrombin time is an excellent marker of liver function over the previous 24 hours. The prothrombin time may also be increased by consumption of clotting factors, as occurs during a massive episode of bleeding.

Protein—a molecule composed of amino acids which generally functions as an enzyme to catalyze a chemical reaction, structural protein or molecular messenger. Hepatitis C contains a number of proteins, including structural core and envelope proteins, as well as enzymes that catalyze replication of the virus.

Pruritus—itching due to liver disease.

Qualitative RNA assay—a test for the presence of hepatitis C RNA in the blood. Results are reported as "positive" or "negative." Usually more sensitive than quantitative hepatitis C RNA assays.

Quantitative RNA assay—a test to determine the quantity of hepatitis C RNA present in the blood. Used to assess response to therapy by measuring a decrease in the amount of RNA present in the bloodstream. Current assays can miss low levels of hepatitis C RNA in the blood.

Rebertron—combination of interferon and ribavirin, marketed by Schering-Plough pharmaceutical company.

Ribavirin—a nucleoside analog or antiviral drug that mimics one of the building blocks of RNA. Shown to have activity against hepatitis C in combination with interferon. The drug's exact mechanism of activity is not well understood. Men and women of childbearing age must both use contraceptives while using this drug and for 6 months after completing treatment. This drug can cause damage to an unborn baby and the birth of a deformed infant.

RIBA—short for recombinant immunoblot assay. Is a more specific method of detecting antibodies to hepatitis C proteins than the EIA test.

RNA—ribonucleic acid. Consists of four nucleotide building blocks strung together in chains of thousands of molecules. Every three nucleotides may code for an amino acid, the building blocks from which proteins are made. Hepatitis C is an RNA virus, which means it carries its genetic information or the instructions on how to make hepatitis C viral proteins in the form of RNA. Hepatitis C RNA circulates in the blood of patients chronically infected with hepatitis C, and this RNA can be tested for in the serum using PCR assays.

Roferon—a brand of interferon manufactured by the Roche Pharmaceuticals Corporation.

Sclerotherapy—a procedure used to obliterate or control bleeding from esophageal varices (engorged blood vessels in the food pipe). Generally involves injecting 5–10 mL fluid into or next to inflamed or bleeding varices. This fluid pushes on the varices and kills adjacent cells, leading to the formation of scar tissue in place of the varices.

SBP—spontaneous bacterial peritonitis. One of the hallmarks of hepatic decompensation, SBP consists of the growth of bacteria in ascitic fluid in the abdomen. Affected people may have increased lassitude or acute abdominal pain and fever. May be insidious in its onset. Treated with antibiotics, SBP is diagnosed by the examination of ascitic fluid for increased white blood cell counts or infectious organisms. Generally viewed as a poor prognostic milestone for patients with end-stage liver disease.

Surgical shunt—portal systemic or distal splenorenal shunts employed to relieve the increased pressure in the vessels draining around the liver, which can lead to variceal bleeding. They involve the surgical grafting of blood vessels from the liver's portal circulation to blood vessels in the systemic circulation which drain back to the heart. Relatively high incidences in postshunt encephalopathy and postsurgical complications has left their application to a highly selected group of patients.

TIPS—transcutaneous interhepatic portal-systemic shunt. A method of relieving the increased pressure in the portal vasculature or major blood vessels feeding into a cirrhotic liver. Generally, this is done to prevent or treat variceal bleeding, but also may be attempted as a technique to treat ascites refractory to medicines.

Transaminases or serum liver enzymes—refers to the liver enzymes commonly referred to AST (SGOT) and ALT (SGPT). The levels of each enzyme are normally detectable in the blood both in sickness and in health. During liver damage or inflammation, these enzymes leak into the bloodstream to higher levels than normal. Patients with hepatitis C are frequently said to have elevated transaminases, or transaminitis.

Wilson's disease—a genetic defect leading to excessive accumulation of copper in the body which can lead to cirrhosis of the liver. Can develop into acute hepatitis in early adulthood. Wilson's disease is diagnosed by liver biopsy and is associated with a low serum ceruloplasmin, hemolysis and neurologic side effects consisting of characteristic jerky muscular movements. Copper-colored rings around the eyes are associated with this condition.

Varices—engorged blood vessels most typically lining the esophagus and stomach that usually develop first in the presence of cirrhosis. They function to carry blood that is no longer able to get through a scarred-up liver as well as it used to. They generally come to attention when there is severe bleeding, often characterized by the emesis, or vomiting, of large quantities of bright red blood all of a sudden. Bleeding varices are a medical emergency and require immediate medical attention.

Virus—a microscopic particle of protein and nucleic acid which enters a cell and produces copies of itself using the cell's metabolic machinery. Hepatitis C is a good example of a virus.

Resource Guide

Alternative Medicine
Several excellent websites are available:
altmed.od.nih.gov/oam/resources/bibs
www.quackwatch.com

Amgen Corporation
Amgen Inc. (Headquarters)
Amgen Center
Thousand Oaks, CA 91320-1789
805/447-1000 (tel)
805/447-1010 (fax)
http://www.AMGEN.com

American Gastroenterological Association (AGA)
Digestive Health Initiative
7910 Woodmont Avenue
Suite 700
Bethesda, MD 20814
http://www.gastro.org/dhi.html

American Association for the Study of Liver Diseases (AASLD)
6900 Grove Road
Thorofare, NJ 08086
http://hepar-sfgh.ucsf.edu/

American Medical Association (AMA)
Healthcare Education Products
515 N. State St.
Chicago, IL 60610
http://www.ama-assn.org

Chiron Corporation
Corporate Communications
4560 Horton Street
Emeryville, CA 94608
510/923-6055
http://www.chiron.com/

Roche Pharmaceuticals
Roche Laboratories
340 Kingsland Street
Nutley, NJ 07110-1199
800/526-6367
800/526-0625
http://www.roche.com/

Schering-Plough Corporation
One Giralda Farms
Madison, NJ 07940-1010
http://www.schering-plough.com

Commitment to Care Program
Assists in finding sources of funding for interferon treatment.
Some "compassionate use" funds available through the
company.
800/521-7157

Be In Charge Program
Provides assistance to organize drug dosing and provides patient education materials, calls from a company-paid "nurse

counselor," support group referrals, therapy management binder, "coaching booklet" for family and friends, side-effects counseling.
888/437-260
www.beincharge.com

American Liver Foundation
1425 Pompton Ave.
Cedar Grove, NJ 07009
Liver disease information hot lines.
800/465-4837
800/443-7222
www.liverfoundation.org

Centers for Disease Control and Prevention
Hepatitis Branch; Mailstop G-37
1600 Clifton Road NE
Atlanta, GA 30333
404/322-4555; 888/4HEPCDC
http://www.cdc.gov/ncidod/disease/hepatitis/C/index.html
http://www.cdc.gov

Hepatitis Foundation International
30 Sunrise Terrace
Cedar Grove, NJ 07009-1423
800/891-0707
http://www.hepfi.org

National Institute of Allergy and Infectious Diseases
Office of Communications
MSC 2520, Bldg. 31, Room 7A50
31 Center Drive
Bethesda, MD 20892-2520
301/496-5717

National Foundation for Infectious Diseases (NFID)
4733 Bethesda Ave., Suite 750
Bethesda, MD 20814
http://www.medscape.com/Affiliates/NFID/

National Digestive Diseases Information Clearinghouse (NDDIC)
2 Information Way
Bethesda, MD 20892-3570
301/654-3810
http://www.niddk.nih.gov

Hepatitis C Foundation
1502 Russett Drive
Warminster, PA 18972
215/672-2606
http://www.hepcfoundation.org

Index

Acknowledgments

I would like to acknowledge my colleagues in the Gastroenterology Division at the University of Michigan as well as hepatologists throughout the country for many insightful discussions; my patients for teaching me so much of this dreaded disease; and the thousands of basic and clinical investigators who helped to develop our knowledge of hepatitis C and its treatments.

I am also forever indebted to Linda Greenspan Regan, executive editor at Plenum Books, for her rapid and expert assistance honing the text to be more easily read both by people infected by hepatitis C and by those interested in learning more about the disease.